Further MCQs in Pharmacy Practice

Further MCQs in Pharmacy Practice

Edited by

Lilian M Azzopardi

BPharm (Hons), MPhil, PhD

Senior Lecturer
Department of Pharmacy
Faculty of Medicine and Surgery
University of Malta
Msida, Malta

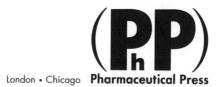

London • Chicago **Pharmaceutical Press**

Published by the Pharmaceutical Press

An imprint of RPS Publishing

1 Lambeth High Street, London SE1 7JN, UK
100 South Atkinson Road, Suite 206, Grayslake, IL 60030-7820, USA

© Pharmaceutical Press 2006

(PhP) is a trade mark of RPS Publishing

RPS Publishing is the publishing organisation of the Royal
Pharmaceutical Society of Great Britain

First published 2006

Typeset by Type Study, Scarborough, North Yorkshire
Printed in Great Britain by TJ International, Padstow, Cornwall

ISBN-10 0 85369 665 9
ISBN-13 978 0 85369 665 0

Contents

Foreword

The role of the pharmacist in counselling patients, other health professionals and the public on the safe, effective and proper use of medications is expanding and has never been more important. At the same time, the knowledge that a pharmacist must have to serve this role is also expanding at an ever-increasing rate. Pharmacists must know, and be able to apply to patient situations, drug and disease information that will allow them to prevent or correct drug overuse, misuse and underuse. The text *Further MCQs in Pharmacy Practice* is targeted towards the needs of final-year pharmacy students and graduates sitting for registration examinations. The format of the text is the presentation of multiple choice questions (MCQs) that address drug and disease knowledge and its application. The questions also test that the pharmacist has a command of the basic knowledge to be able to carry out the services in an intelligent way. Questions addressing pharmaceutical calculations, formulations, medicinal chemistry and pathology are included. There is both an open-book section of questions and a closed-book section. For each answer there is an explanatory section, indicating why the selected answer is correct or incorrect. The present text is an extension of the publication by Dr Azzopardi and colleagues entitled *MCQs in Pharmacy Practice*, which was published in 2003. The questions cover a wide range of therapeutic areas. The MCQs take different formats to challenge one's knowledge in a variety of ways. In my estimation, *Further MCQs in Pharmacy Practice* should prove to be very valuable to pharmacy students and graduates seeking registration in allowing a careful self-assessment of their drug and disease knowledge. The information covered in the questions is comprehensive and very relevant to pharmacy practice. The open-book section and the provision of explanations to the answers will help the reader identify areas of strengths and weaknesses in pharmacy knowledge and where to spend additional reading and review time. Of note, practising pharmacists would also likely benefit from a self-assessment through *Further MCQs in Pharmacy Practice* to contribute to their continuing professional development. I highly recommend the text and commend the authors for providing a practical and useful educational tool for self-assessment of drug and disease knowledge that is pertinent to pharmacy practice.

Peter H Vlasses, PharmD, BCPS, FCCP
Executive Director
Accreditation Council for Pharmacy Education (ACPE)
Chicago, Illinois, USA
June 2006

Preface

Pharmacy educators have a responsibility towards society to ensure that pharmacy graduates have the skills to practise the profession competently. During pharmacy education, assessments are carried out over the years to develop a graduate's portfolio, which demonstrates the ability of the graduates to perform the different skills. For a graduate to be able to practise the profession competently, assessments are carried out to evaluate the development of a knowledge base, the interpretation and application of knowledge, evaluation of data, mathematical skills and time management. To be able to achieve this, pharmacy education systems should ensure that a programme of education and training is provided to graduates who will be able to reach these goals. During the 2005 Annual Conference of the European Association of Faculties of Pharmacy (EAFP), the Malta Declaration on pharmacy education was adopted by the Executive Committee and delegates from 68 schools of pharmacy and pharmacy institutions from 29 countries. The scope of the EAFP Malta Declaration is to define university courses for pharmacy education programmes so as to promote harmonisation and cooperation among faculties of pharmacy in Europe. This will promote international student and staff mobility and supports recognition of professional qualifications between member states of the European Union. EAFP holds that pharmacist education programmes should be equivalent to at least 300 ECTS. A balance between theoretical, laboratory and patient centred training is required while maintaining the university character of the curriculum. A thorough grounding in the basic sciences, including research approach, should be maintained while contemporary developments in pharmacy namely pharmaceutical care, professionalism-values, behaviours and attitudes, clinical pharmacy and clinical analysis, prescription and non-prescription medicines regulatory affairs, pharmacoeconomics, medical devices and industrial pharmacy should be given adequate coverage. A six-month traineeship in a pharmacy that is open to the public or in a hospital under the supervision of a pharmacist should be carried out within the university course so as to integrate the knowledge base and professional practice within a university milieu. In addition, training periods should also be considered during the course for other pharmacy-related areas such as industrial pharmacy. Training periods may also be offered in one or more optional areas, depending on the individual institution. EAFP recommends at least a five-year programme of university education and training for a pharmacist to ensure that the individual has acquired knowledge and skills in the scientific areas of chemistry and manufacture of medicines, effects, actions and use of medicines as well as in the practice areas of the provision of professional services according to good professional standards, evaluation of information on medicines and pursuit of continuing professional development programmes in the interest of patients requiring therapeutical intervention. This declaration outlines a framework that may be followed by schools of pharmacy to ensure a sound development of the graduates' portfolio. The students should ensure that they are able to demonstrate that they have developed the necessary skills to practise the profession competently. By using textbooks such as *Further MCQs in Pharmacy Practice*, prepared by Lilian M. Azzopardi and her colleagues, the students have a useful tool, which helps them to undertake self-assessment procedures. Self-assessment is a healthy way to study and prepare for final examinations and registration examinations. With the explanations provided and the data presented in the appendices, pharmacy students should be able to use this book as a useful revision aid prior to assessments.

Professor Benito del Castillo Garcia
Dean, Faculty of Pharmacy
University Complutense, Madrid, Spain
President, European Association of Faculties of Pharmacy
June 2006

Introduction

A number of pharmacy examination boards who act as the final judges in allowing a candidate to practise unsupervised as a pharmacist are using multiple choice questions (MCQs) as a useful tool to help them in making their decision. This not only applies to pharmacy, and MCQs are now commonly used to examine several other healthcare professionals.

The responsibility in formulating these examination questions is significant. While there is a requirement to ensure that candidates who present a threat to pharmacy practice are identified, thus ensuring that they should not obtain a pass mark in the examination, the examination should also ensure that competent candidates do make the grade.

The same principles that are used for making up questions for examinations were used in preparing this book. The questions set in this book have all been analysed and considered valid and satisfactory. The book is a continuation of a previous publication that was very well received. All the questions are new cases covering traditional areas while some other topics, which have recently received greater attention in pharmacy practice, are also included. The book takes the form of test papers consisting of a number of questions taken from actual tests undertaken by pharmacy students who have followed a five-year course of studies and practice. The results obtained by these students for tests 1 to 6 are shown in Appendix D.

MCQ examinations frequently present a problem to prospective candidates in how to prepare for them, as opposed to the more traditional essay type or problem type exams. It is not realistic to expect candidates to memorise whole sections of reference books such as the *British National Formulary*, nor is it feasible for students to anticipate with what questions they are likely to be faced. For this reason, the examiners frequently include two types of questions; those that the candidates will be expected to answer from their own knowledge and experience without reference to any text, the closed-book questions, and others that the candidate is expected to answer by referring to standard sources that the professional would be expected to have available during practice, the open-book questions.

The profession of pharmacy is based on science and practice. The questions in a comprehensive examination aim to reflect this. In practice both generic and proprietary names are encountered. Pharmacists must be familiar with both.

By going through the questions posed in this book and considering the rationale for the answers given at the end, the candidate will gain a useful insight as to what might be expected in the actual examination and thus be better prepared for it.

Acknowledgements

I would like to thank a number of colleagues who have assisted me in one way or another in the preparation of this publication. In particular I would like to express my thanks to Professor Anthony Serracino-Inglott, Head of Department of Pharmacy at the University of Malta and Dr Maurice Zarb-Adami for their contributions towards the book. Their knowledge and hands-on experience in pharmacy education has added greatly to the robustness of the book. I also would like to thank Professor Steve Hudson, University of Strathclyde, Dr Sam Salek, University of Cardiff and Professor Vincenzo Tortorella, University of Bari for their contributions and for the good times we shared during the discussions we had in preparation for the book. In addition I would like to thank Professor Victor Ferrito, University of Malta for reviewing material in the book.

My sincere thanks go to Professor Roger Ellul-Micallef, Rector, and Professor Godfrey LaFerla, Dean of the Faculty of Medicine and Surgery of the University of Malta for their support and encouragement. I would also like to thank Peter Vlasses, Executive Director, Accreditation Council for Pharmacy Education, USA and Professor Benito del Castillo Garcia, University Complutense Madrid for their interest in the publication.

I would like to acknowledge the support of my colleagues and the staff at the Department of Pharmacy and the Faculty of Medicine and Surgery of the University of Malta. I would like to mention the pharmacy students at the Department of Pharmacy and colleagues from different countries for their comments on *MCQs in Pharmacy Practice*. Their comments and positive feedback gave us the encouragement to prepare this publication. Thanks also go to the staff at the Pharmaceutical Press for their work in the preparation and production of this publication.

Special thanks to my sister Louise, a clinical pharmacist, for her much appreciated comments and valuable suggestions. Finally, I would like to thank my family and friends for their interest and encouragement throughout the preparation of the book.

About the editor

Lilian M Azzopardi studied pharmacy at the University of Malta, Faculty of Medicine and Surgery. In 1994 she took up a position at the Department of Pharmacy, University of Malta as a teaching and research assistant. Dr Azzopardi began an MPhil on the development of formulary systems for community pharmacy, which was completed in 1995, and in 1999 she completed a PhD which led to the publication of the book *Validation Instruments for Community Pharmacy: Pharmaceutical Care for the Third Millennium* published in 2000 by Pharmaceutical Products Press, USA. She worked together with Professor Anthony Serracino Inglott who was a pioneer in the introduction of clinical pharmacy in the late 60s. In 2003 Dr Azzopardi edited the book *MCQs in Pharmacy Practice* published by the Pharmaceutical Press, UK.

Throughout her career Lilian M Azzopardi has been actively involved in pharmacy practice teaching and in research in pharmacy practice. She is currently a senior lecturer in pharmacy practice at the Department of Pharmacy, University of Malta and is responsible for co-ordinating the teaching of pharmacy practice, including the planning, organisation and assessment of pharmacy practice during the undergraduate course as well as during the preregistration period. Dr Azzopardi is an examiner in pharmacy practice and clinical pharmacy for the course of pharmacy at the University of Malta.

Lilian Azzopardi was for a short period interim director of the European Society of Clinical Pharmacy (ESCP) and is currently coordinator of the ESCP newsletter. She served as a member of the Working Group on Quality Care Standards within the Community Pharmacy Section of the International Pharmaceutical Federation (FIP). In 1997 she received an award from the FIP Foundation for Education and Research and in 1999 was awarded the ESCP German Research and Education Foundation grant.

Lilian Azzopardi has published several papers on clinical pharmacy and pharmaceutical care and has actively participated at congresses organised by FIP, ESCP, the Royal Pharmaceutical Society of Great Britain, the American Pharmaceutical Association and the American Society of Health-System Pharmacists. In 2002 Dr Azzopardi was invited to contribute to the first sessions of compulsory continuing professional development programme for pharmacists in Italy.

Contributors

Lilian M Azzopardi BPharm(Hons), MPhil, PhD
Senior Lecturer, Department of Pharmacy, University of Malta, Msida, Malta

Stephen A Hudson MPharm, FRPharmS
Professor of Pharmaceutical Care, Division of Pharmaceutical Sciences, Strathclyde Institute of Pharmacy and Biomedical Sciences, University of Strathclyde, Glasgow, UK

Sam Salek BPharm, PhD, RPh, MFPM(Hon)
Professor and Director, Centre for Socioeconomic Research, Welsh School of Pharmacy, Cardiff, UK

Anthony Serracino-Inglott BPharm, PharmD
Professor and Head of Department, Department of Pharmacy, University of Malta, Msida, Malta

Vincenzo Tortorella PhD, DIC(Lond)
Professor and Dean, Faculty of Pharmacy, University of Bari, Bari, Italy

Maurice Zarb Adami BPharm, PhD
Senior Lecturer, Department of Pharmacy, University of Malta, Msida, Malta

How to use

The questions are divided into sets of an open-book and of a closed-book type. Each test consists of 100 questions and there are a total of six tests and therefore 600 questions. In addition another 10 questions have been grouped in Test 7 to introduce readers to a format of MCQs that is becoming more popular with time. They are referred to as MCQs in a sequential format. In this case the candidate is presented with a number of proposed answers which have a different probability of being correct. The candidate has to list the given answers according to the relative probability of being correct. The questions in Test 7 are also unique in that they deal with the application of basic sciences to practice, an area that did not feature prominently in Tests 1 to 6.

You should tackle all the questions in one test in one session, and write down the answer on a sheet of paper, as though under examination conditions, namely, using or refraining from using reference texts as the case may be.

Make a note of the time it takes to cover each test, so that these may be added up at the end to allow you to pace yourself. The answers for the tests can then be compared with the answers given in the book. You will thus start to gain some intuition or feeling into the examiners' thinking and logic in setting particular questions. This should help in addressing the other sections, and in the end, the actual examination itself.

Keep in mind that each question carries a particular mark, and this cannot be exceeded even if you spend extra time on it. On the other hand, some questions are quite straightforward, and marks allotted to such questions should not be missed.

When all the tests have been covered in the way suggested above, examine the explanatory notes at the end to see whether the difficulties that you encountered are also commonly met by other students.

Revision checklist

For each test, write the number of the question and your answer on a separate sheet of paper then, after going through all the questions in the test, compare your answers with those in the book.

Refer to Appendix D for feedback on those questions that you did not answer correctly to be able to compare your ability with a cohort of students.

You can obtain information on the proprietary names listed in the book in Appendix A. Appendix B includes definitions for medical terms included in the book while Appendix C lists abbreviations and acronyms.

Recommended textbooks for the open-book section are:

Azzopardi LM (2000). *Validation Instruments for Community Pharmacy: Pharmaceutical Care for the Third Millennium*, Binghamton, New York: Pharmaceutical Products Press.

Edwards C, Stillman P (2006). *Minor Illness or Major Disease? Responding to Symptoms in the Pharmacy*, 4th edn. London: Pharmaceutical Press.

Harman RJ, Mason P, eds (2002). *Handbook of Pharmacy Healthcare: Diseases and Patient Advice*, 2nd edn. London: Pharmaceutical Press.

Mehta DK, ed (2006). *British National Formulary*, 51st edn. London: Pharmaceutical Press.

Nathan A (2002). *Non-prescription Medicines*, 2nd edn. London: Pharmaceutical Press.

Royal Pharmaceutical Society of Great Britain (2005). *Medicines, Ethics and Practice: a Guide for Pharmacists*. London: Pharmaceutical Press.

Checklist

This checklist should help students identify areas that need to be covered when preparing for comprehensive final examinations and preregistration exams.

- *Action and use of drugs:* classification, medicinal chemistry, mechanism of action, pharmacokinetics, dosage regimen, patient monitoring, patient counselling, cautionary labels
- *Responding to symptoms:* presentation of conditions, diagnosis, referrals, use of non-prescription medicines, patient counselling
- *Adverse effects:* common adverse effects, patient counselling, patient monitoring
- *Cautions and contraindications:* disease states, baseline tests required
- *Special requirements:* dose adjustments in liver and hepatic disease, use of drugs during pregnancy and breast-feeding, geriatric and paediatric patients, palliative care
- *Diagnostics:* medical devices, point-of-care tests, interpretation of results
- *Calculations:* dose calculations, dilutions
- *Health promotion and disease prevention:* lifestyle and dietary modifications, prophylaxis against disease
- *Standards of practice:* evaluation methods, audit processes, management, documentation, quality assurance, operating procedures

Section 1

Open-book questions

Test 1

Questions

Questions 1–10

Directions: Each of the questions or incomplete statements is followed by five suggested answers. Select the best answer in each case.

Q1 All the following products used in the treatment of glaucoma are applied topically EXCEPT:

A ☐ Xalatan
B ☐ Diamox
C ☐ Trusopt
D ☐ Timoptol
E ☐ Betoptic

Q2 Which is an alternative preparation of Lipitor?

A ☐ Cozaar
B ☐ Lescol
C ☐ Zestril
D ☐ Cardura
E ☐ Trandate

Q3 Tambocor:

A ☐ may be of value in serious symptomatic ventricular arrhythmias
B ☐ is a beta-adrenoceptor blocker
C ☐ is available only for parenteral administration
D ☐ cannot be administered concurrently with antibacterial agents
E ☐ is a proprietary preparation for amiodarone

Q4 Terazosin:

A ☐ constricts smooth muscle
B ☐ is a selective beta-blocker
C ☐ increases urinary flow rate
D ☐ may cause an increase in blood pressure
E ☐ is indicated in urinary frequency

Q5 Legionnaires' disease:

A ☐ is caused by a Gram-positive coccus
B ☐ is a chronic infectious disease
C ☐ has an incubation period of 2 days to 3 years
D ☐ is characterised by the development of pneumonia
E ☐ may be prevented by vaccination

Q6 Trigger factors for migraine include all EXCEPT:

A ☐ use of caffeine
B ☐ exposure to sunlight
C ☐ missed meals
D ☐ lack of sleep
E ☐ air travel

Q7 All the following products contain a local anaesthetic EXCEPT:

A ☐ Dequacaine
B ☐ Merocaine
C ☐ BurnEze
D ☐ Anthisan
E ☐ Proctosedyl

Q8 Good pharmacy practice guidelines:

A ☐ have been established by the International Pharmaceutical Federation (FIP)
B ☐ comply with ISO 9000
C ☐ consist of an audit process
D ☐ relate to pharmaceutical marketing
E ☐ entail field observation studies

Q9 Anti-D immunoglobulin:

A ☐ is available as oral tablets
B ☐ is a vaccination for tetanus
C ☐ should be administered preferably within 72 h of a sensitising episode
D ☐ is intended to protect the mother from haemolytic disease
E ☐ cannot be used for prophylaxis

Q10 Which of the following products is NOT indicated for the management of peptic ulceration?

A ☐ Zantac
B ☐ Gaviscon
C ☐ Nexium
D ☐ Pariet
E ☐ Buscopan

Questions 11–34

Directions: Each group of questions below consists of five lettered headings followed by a list of numbered questions. For each numbered question select the one heading that is most closely related to it. Each heading may be used once, more than once or not at all.

Questions 11–13 concern the following drugs:

A ☐ valaciclovir
B ☐ griseofulvin
C ☐ itraconazole
D ☐ famciclovir
E ☐ terbinafine

Select, from A to E, which one of the above corresponds to the brand name:

Q11 Famvir

Q12 Sporanox

Q13 Lamisil

Questions 14–17 concern the following drugs:

A ☐ nalidixic acid
B ☐ norfloxacin
C ☐ levofloxacin
D ☐ ofloxacin
E ☐ amphotericin

Select, from A to E, which one of the above:

Q14 can be used for intestinal candidiasis

Q15 has greater activity than ciprofloxacin against pneumococci

Q16 is marketed as Tavanic

Q17   is only indicated in urinary tract infection

Questions 18–20 concern the following drugs:

A   ☐   atenolol
B   ☐   folic acid
C   ☐   imipramine
D   ☐   carbamazepine
E   ☐   co-trimoxazole

Select, from A to E, during pregnancy which one of the above:

Q18   may cause intrauterine growth restriction

Q19   may increase the risk of neural tube defects

Q20   may increase the risk of tachycardia in neonate

Questions 21–23 concern the following maximum oral daily doses:

A   ☐   200 mg daily
B   ☐   150 mg daily
C   ☐   100 mg daily
D   ☐   50 mg daily
E   ☐   300 mg daily

Select, from A to E, which one of the above corresponds to:

Q21   diclofenac

Q22   sildenafil

Q23   sumatriptan

Questions 24–26 concern the following cautionary labels:

A ☐ To be sucked or chewed.

B ☐ With or after food.

C ☐ Follow the printed instructions you have been given with this medicine.

D ☐ Avoid exposure of skin to direct sunlight or sun lamps.

E ☐ Do not stop taking this medicine except on your doctor's advice.

Select, from A to E, which one of the above corresponds to the drugs:

Q24 chlorpromazine

Q25 dapsone

Q26 warfarin

Questions 27–30 concern the following products:

A ☐ AeroChamber

B ☐ Nuelin

C ☐ Atrovent

D ☐ Beconase

E ☐ Alupent

Select, from A to E, which one of the above corresponds to the following presentations:

Q27 syrup

Q28 aerosol for inhalation

Q29 spacer device

Q30 nasal spray

Questions 31–34 concern the following tablet descriptions:

A   ☐ yellow 40 mg
B   ☐ brown 1 mg
C   ☐ yellow 250 mg
D   ☐ red-brown 100 mg
E   ☐ yellow 2.5 mg

Select, from A to E, which one of the above corresponds to the following preparations:

Q31   Klaricid

Q32   Diovan

Q33   warfarin

Q34   Zomig

Questions 35–60

Directions: For each of the questions below, ONE or MORE of the responses is (are) correct. Decide which of the responses is (are) correct. Then choose:

A   ☐ if 1, 2 and 3 are correct
B   ☐ if 1 and 2 only are correct
C   ☐ if 2 and 3 only are correct
D   ☐ if 1 only is correct
E   ☐ if 3 only is correct

Directions summarised				
A	**B**	**C**	**D**	**E**
1, 2, 3	1, 2 only	2, 3 only	1 only	3 only

Q35 When administering cisplatin powder for injection:

1 ☐ it should be reconstituted with water for injection
2 ☐ it should be given over 6–8 h
3 ☐ the infusion fluid used is Ringer's solution

Q36 Ceftazidime:

1 ☐ is a 'third-generation' cephalosporin antibacterial
2 ☐ is more active than cefuroxime against Gram-positive bacteria
3 ☐ is available as tablets and injections

Q37 Potentially hazardous interactions could occur between:

1 ☐ ergotamine and zolmitriptan
2 ☐ warfarin and gliclazide
3 ☐ combined oral contraceptives and clindamycin

Q38 Examples of enzyme inducers include:

1 ☐ griseofulvin
2 ☐ rifampicin
3 ☐ warfarin

Q39 Which of the following drugs may be used in patients with liver disease but require a dose reduction?

1 ☐ Natrilix
2 ☐ Nizoral
3 ☐ Zyloric

Q40 Capsulitis:

1 ☐ is a disorder affecting the shoulder
2 ☐ may be caused by unaccustomed movement
3 ☐ is an inflammatory process

Q41 Presentations of a facial lesion that warrant referral include:

1 ☐ swollen lymph glands in the neck
2 ☐ butterfly distribution of a rash over the nose and cheeks
3 ☐ a scaly rash with mild erythema affecting the forehead and eyebrows

Q42 Antacid preparations containing sodium bicarbonate include:

1 ☐ Gaviscon liquid
2 ☐ Bisodol Heartburn Relief tablets
3 ☐ Maalox Plus tablets

Q43 The agents associated with pain and inflammation of a bee sting include:

1 ☐ histamine
2 ☐ apamin
3 ☐ hyaluronidase

Q44 Antispasmodics that could be recommended for irritable bowel syndrome include:

1 ☐ Colofac
2 ☐ Spasmonal
3 ☐ Fybogel

Q45 Paradichlorobenzene:

1 ☐ has antifungal properties
2 ☐ is used as a disinfectant
3 ☐ is present in Cerumol drops

Q46   Aspirin:

1   ☐ potentiates the anticoagulant effect of warfarin
2   ☐ inhibits platelet aggregation
3   ☐ promotes vitamin K synthesis

Q47   Male pattern baldness:

1   ☐ is androgenetic alopecia
2   ☐ is caused by the release of prostaglandins
3   ☐ may be precipitated by chemical hair preparations

Q48   Finasteride:

1   ☐ is an enzyme inhibitor
2   ☐ is an anti-androgen
3   ☐ could be used in male-pattern baldness

Q49   Diamorphine:

1   ☐ is a controlled drug
2   ☐ is more lipid soluble than morphine
3   ☐ may be administered intramuscularly

Q50   Drugs that could be used in nausea and vomiting caused by palliative cancer treatment include:

1   ☐ metoclopramide
2   ☐ haloperidol
3   ☐ prochlorperazine

Q51   Bacterial conjunctivitis:

1   ❏ is an infectious condition
2   ❏ affects both eyes
3   ❏ is associated with pain

Q52   Wet skin lesions:

1   ❏ indicate presence of a fungal infection
2   ❏ always require referral
3   ❏ potassium permanganate soaks may be recommended

Q53   Infant formula milk preparations:

1   ❏ may be based on cow's milk
2   ❏ contain no fat
3   ❏ are presented as separate components to be reconstituted before use

Q54   Staphylococcal napkin dermatitis:

1   ❏ occurs when the patient also has oral thrush
2   ❏ presents as a pustular rash
3   ❏ should be referred

Q55   Sialolithiasis:

1   ❏ is the inflammation of a salivary gland
2   ❏ presents with facial pain and swelling
3   ❏ is associated with eating

Q56 Accompanying conditions that require referral when patients present with ear problems include:

1 ☐ history of perforated ear drum
2 ☐ discharge
3 ☐ pain

Q57 When patients present with complaints related to indigestion the pharmacist should enquire whether:

1 ☐ symptoms are related to food intake patterns
2 ☐ accompanying symptoms include vomiting or constipation
3 ☐ the patient is wheezing

Q58 Kaolin and Morphine Mixture:

1 ☐ is not recommended for acute diarrhoea
2 ☐ contains a low concentration of morphine
3 ☐ contains kaolin, which may reduce bioavailability of morphine

Q59 Meggezones pastilles:

1 ☐ contain pseudoephedrine
2 ☐ provide a soothing effect through the promotion of saliva production
3 ☐ should not be recommended to diabetic patients

Q60 In migraine:

1 ☐ a soluble oral drug formulation is preferred to a solid oral dosage form
2 ☐ an analgesic should be taken at the first sign of an attack
3 ☐ Syndol may be recommended

Questions 61–80

Directions: The following questions consist of a first statement followed by a second statement. Decide whether the first statement is true or false. Decide whether the second statement is true or false. Then choose:

A   ❑ if both statements are true and the second statement is a **correct explanation** of the first statement

B   ❑ if both statements are true but the second statement **is NOT a correct explanation** of the first statement

C   ❑ if the first statement is true but the second statement is false

D   ❑ if the first statement is false but the second statement is true

E   ❑ if both statements are false

Directions summarised			
	First statement	**Second statement**	
A	True	True	Second statement is a *correct explanation* of the first
B	True	True	Second statement is *NOT a correct explanation* of the first
C	True	False	
D	False	True	
E	False	False	

Q61   Hydroxychloroquine is used to treat rheumatoid arthritis. Hydroxychloroquine is better tolerated than gold.

Q62   Acute attacks of porphyria may be precipitated by drug administration. Progestogen-containing preparations should be avoided in patients with porphyria.

Q63   Goserelin may be used in prostrate cancer. Goserelin may result in a tumour 'flare'.

Q64 Tacrolimus is chemically similar to ciclosporin. Tacrolimus has a similar mode of action to ciclosporin.

Q65 In older patients, imipramine may cause hyponatraemia. Hyponatraemia occurs because of increased sodium re-uptake in the loop of Henle.

Q66 Inflammation of the larynx requires the administration of atropine. Atropine is a sympathomimetic agent.

Q67 Lidocaine is used in ventricular arrhythmias. Lidocaine suppresses ventricular tachycardia and reduces the risk of ventricular fibrillation following myocardial infarction.

Q68 Propranolol is preferred to atenolol in hypertensive patients with moderate kidney damage. Propranolol is not water soluble and is not excreted by the kidneys.

Q69 Filgrastim is used for neutropenia induced by cytotoxic chemotherapy. Filgrastim is an example of a recombinant human erythropoietin.

Q70 Intake of drugs at therapeutic doses in mothers who are breast-feeding are not likely to cause toxicity in the infant. Toxicity in the infant always occurs when the drug enters the milk.

Q71 Pemphigus is an autoimmune reaction. Immunosuppressants such as ciclosporin are the first line of treatment in pemphigus.

Q72 Ear pain during air travel occurs because of a problem in the external ear. Nasal decongestants may be used to prevent this condition.

Q73 Agranulocytosis could occur as a result of Stelazine therapy. Stelazine is trimipramine.

Q74 Tinnitus may be an adverse effect of furosemide. All diuretics may cause tinnitus.

Q75 Concomitant use of St John's wort and sertraline should be avoided. St John's wort is used for mild depression.

Q76 Co-codamol preparations that can be sold over-the-counter contain codeine 60 mg. Co-codamol is a combination of codeine and dextropropoxyphene.

Q77 Varicella is a highly contagious disease. Prophylaxis for varicella is not available.

Q78 Graduated compression hosiery should not be used during pregnancy. Graduated compression hosiery prevents oedema.

Q79 First-line treatment of nocturnal enuresis is drug treatment. Amitriptyline may be used in nocturnal enuresis.

Q80 Betahistine is indicated for motion sickness. Betahistine may be associated with headache.

Questions 81–100

Directions: These questions involve prescriptions or patient requests. Read the prescription or patient request and answer the questions.

Questions 81–85: Use the prescription below:

Patient's name   ....
Premarin 0.625 mg tablets
1 od   m 28
Doctor's signature   ....

Q81   Premarin contains

A   ☐ conjugated oestrogens 625 µg
B   ☐ conjugated oestrogens 62.5 µg
C   ☐ conjugated oestrogens 0.625 µg
D   ☐ conjugated oestrogens 625 µg and levonorgestrel 75 µg
E   ☐ conjugated oestrogens 0.625 µg and levonorgestrel 75 µg

Q82   Premarin is also available as:

1   ☐ a nasal spray
2   ☐ patches
3   ☐ tablets in a different strength

A   ☐ 1, 2, 3
B   ☐ 1, 2 only
C   ☐ 2, 3 only
D   ☐ 1 only
E   ☐ 3 only

Q83   Premarin:

1   ☐ is indicated in women with an intact uterus
2   ☐ may be used for prophylaxis of osteoporosis
3   ☐ is marketed by Wyeth

A   ☐ 1, 2, 3
B   ☐ 1, 2 only
C   ☐ 2, 3 only
D   ☐ 1 only
E   ☐ 3 only

Q84   An equivalent product to Premarin is:

A   ☐   Nuvelle
B   ☐   Progynova
C   ☐   Trisequens
D   ☐   Prempak-C
E   ☐   Femoston

Q85   The patient should:

1   ☐   take one Premarin tablet daily
2   ☐   take tablets for 28 days followed by a 7-day break before starting the next pack
3   ☐   undertake regular visits to a general practitioner every 15 days

A   ☐   1, 2, 3
B   ☐   1, 2 only
C   ☐   2, 3 only
D   ☐   1 only
E   ☐   3 only

Questions 86–87: Use the prescription below:

Patient's name   ....

Fosamax tablets
70 mg once per week

Doctor's signature   ....

Q86   Fosamax:

A   ☐ contains disodium etidronate
B   ☐ increases rate of bone turnover
C   ☐ may cause dysphagia
D   ☐ can impair bone mineralisation
E   ☐ acts as a posterior pituitary hormone antagonist

Q87   Fosamax:

1   ☐ a weekly treatment costs about £6
2   ☐ is available only as 5 mg tablets
3   ☐ the patient has to take three tablets weekly

A   ☐ 1, 2, 3
B   ☐ 1, 2 only
C   ☐ 2, 3 only
D   ☐ 1 only
E   ☐ 3 only

Questions 88–90: Use the prescription below:

Patient's name   ....
Combivent
2 puffs qds
Doctor's signature   ....

Q88   Combivent consists of:

1   ❏ ipratropium
2   ❏ salbutamol
3   ❏ salmeterol

A   ❏ 1, 2, 3
B   ❏ 1, 2 only
C   ❏ 2, 3 only
D   ❏ 1 only
E   ❏ 3 only

Q89   Combivent is available as:

1   ❏ dry powder for inhalation
2   ❏ a nebuliser solution
3   ❏ an aerosol inhalation

A   ❏ 1, 2, 3
B   ❏ 1, 2 only
C   ❏ 2, 3 only
D   ❏ 1 only
E   ❏ 3 only

Q90   Combivent is not available. Which of the following products could be recommended to replace Combivent?

1   ❏ Ventolin
2   ❏ Atrovent
3   ❏ Becotide

A   ❏ 1, 2, 3
B   ❏ 1, 2 only
C   ❏ 2, 3 only
D   ❏ 1 only
E   ❏ 3 only

Questions 91–92: Use the prescription below:

Patient's name   ....

Depo-Medrone
m 1

Doctor's signature   ....

Q91   Depo-Medrone:

1   ☐   consists of methylprednisolone
2   ☐   is used to suppress an allergic reaction
3   ☐   may be used in rheumatic disease

A   ☐   1, 2, 3
B   ☐   1, 2 only
C   ☐   2, 3 only
D   ☐   1 only
E   ☐   3 only

Q92   Depo-Medrone:

1   ☐   is administered parenterally
2   ☐   may be administered twice daily
3   ☐   is highly likely to cause cerebral oedema

A   ☐   1, 2, 3
B   ☐   1, 2 only
C   ☐   2, 3 only
D   ☐   1 only
E   ☐   3 only

Questions 93–96: Use the prescription below:

Patient's name ....
Persantin Retard
1 bd   m 60
Aspirin 75 mg
1 daily   m 60
Doctor's signature ....

Q93 Persantin Retard is an:

A ☐ anticoagulant
B ☐ antiplatelet
C ☐ analgesic
D ☐ antihypertensive
E ☐ anti-arrhythmic drug

Q94 The side-effects that could occur with Persantin Retard include:

1 ☐ gastrointestinal effects
2 ☐ worsening of symptoms of coronary heart disease
3 ☐ hot flushes

A ☐ 1, 2, 3
B ☐ 1, 2 only
C ☐ 2, 3 only
D ☐ 1 only
E ☐ 3 only

Q95 The pharmacist should dispense Persantin Retard in its original container because:

A ☐ the pack also includes aspirin
B ☐ the original pack is better labelled
C ☐ such dispensing saves time in counting capsules
D ☐ the original pack contains a dessicant
E ☐ it is a controlled drug

Q96 Regarding the Persantin Retard, the patient is instructed to:

A ☐ take two capsules together at breakfast
B ☐ discard any capsules remaining 6 weeks after opening
C ☐ double the dose before undergoing surgery
D ☐ abstain from driving when taking these medications
E ☐ keep the medicines prescribed in a refrigerator

Questions 97–100: For each question read the patient request:

Q97 A parent requests a multivitamin preparation for a 6-year-old child. Which product could be recommended?

A ☐ Forceval
B ☐ Vivioptal
C ☐ Maxepa
D ☐ En-De-Kay
E ☐ Calcium-Sandoz

Q98 A mother requests a preparation for her 5-year-old son for a chesty cough. Which of the following products is the most appropriate?

A ☐ Benylin with Codeine syrup

B ☐ Alupent syrup

C ☐ Actifed Chesty Coughs syrup

D ☐ Vicks Medinite syrup

E ☐ Neoclarityn syrup

Q99 A patient asks for ibuprofen gel. The pharmacist may dispense:

A ☐ Oruvail

B ☐ Voltarol

C ☐ Dubam

D ☐ Brufen

E ☐ Ibutop

Q100 A patient asks for a preparation as a vaginal cream for candidiasis. Which product is the most appropriate?

A ☐ Canesten

B ☐ Ortho-Gynest

C ☐ Eurax

D ☐ Bactroban

E ☐ Dermovate

Test 1

Answers

A1   B

Diamox contains acetazolamide, which is a carbonic anhydrase inhibitor administered orally or by the parenteral route. Xalatan contains latanoprost, a prostaglandin analogue, and Trusopt contains dorzolamide, a carbonic anhydrase inhibitor. Timoptol and Betoptic both consist of beta-blockers containing timolol and betaxolol respectively.

A2   B

Lipitor contains atorvastatin. An alternative preparation is Lescol, which contains another statin, fluvastatin. Cozaar contains losartan, an angiotensin-II receptor antagonist, Zestril contains lisinopril, an angiotensin-converting enzyme inhibitor, Cardura contains doxazosin, an alpha-adrenoceptor blocking drug, and Trandate contains labetalol, a beta-adrenoceptor blocking drug.

A3   A

Tambocor contains flecainide, which may be of value in serious symptomatic ventricular arrhythmias. It is also indicated for junctional re-entry tachycardias and for paroxysmal atrial fibrillation. It is available as tablets or injections for intravenous administration. Hazardous interactions may be expected when flecainide is administered concurrently with drugs such as amiodarone, tricyclic antidepressants, terfenadine, ritonavir, dolasetron, clozapine, verapamil, and with beta-blockers. Amiodarone is a drug that is also indicated in the treatment of arrhythmias. An example of a proprietary name for amiodarone is Cordarone X.

A4 C

Terazosin is a selective alpha-blocker that relaxes smooth muscle and is indicated in benign prostatic hyperplasia because it increases urinary flow rate and improves obstructive symptoms. Terazosin is also indicated in the management of mild-to-moderate hypertension. After the first dose a rapid reduction in blood pressure may occur.

A5 D

Legionnaires' disease is an acute respiratory tract infection caused by a Gram-negative bacillus of the *Legionella* species. It is characterised by the development of pneumonia. The incubation period is from 2 to 10 days. The condition is attributed to the inhalation of water droplets, such as from water generated in air-conditioning cooling systems and in hot-water systems, that are contaminated with the microorganism. Prevention techniques are based on the maintenance of air-conditioning filters and water systems.

A6 D

Trigger factors for migraine include intake of specific food such as caffeine, chocolate, cheese and alcoholic drinks, exposure to light, hunger and missed meals, and air travel.

A7 D

Anthisan contains mepyramine, an antihistamine. Dequacaine contains benzocaine and dequalinium, Merocaine contains benzocaine and cetylpyridinium, BurnEze contains benzocaine, and Proctosedyl contains cinchocaine and hydrocortisone. Benzocaine and cinchocaine are anaesthetics.

A8 A

During the FIP congress in Japan in 1993 the international guidelines for *Good Pharmacy Practice* (GPP) were adopted. A revised version of these guidelines,

Standards for Quality of Pharmacy Services, was endorsed during the 35th meeting of the World Health Organization's Expert Committee on Specifications for Pharmaceutical Preparations in April 1997 and this was approved by the FIP Congress in Vancouver in 1997.

A9   C

Anti-D(Rh$_0$) immunoglobulin should be administered immediately or within 72 h of any sensitising episode during abortion, miscarriage or giving birth to a rhesus-positive foetus. It prevents a rhesus-negative mother from forming antibodies to rhesus-positive cells that may pass into the maternal circulation. It is intended to protect any subsequent child from haemolytic disease. It is available as an injection.

A10   E

Buscopan contains hyoscine, which is a quaternary ammonium compound having antimuscarinic activity. It is indicated for symptomatic relief of gastrointestinal or genitourinary disorders characterised by smooth muscle spasm. Zantac contains ranitidine, which is an H$_2$-receptor antagonist that promotes healing of peptic ulcers by reducing gastric output as a result of histamine H$_2$-receptor blockade. Nexium contains esomeprazole and Pariet contains rabeprazole, both of which are proton pump inhibitors. The proton pump inhibitors inhibit gastric acid output by blocking the hydrogen–potassium–adenosine triphosphatase enzyme system of the gastric parietal cells. Gaviscon is an antacid preparation that can be used for the management of symptoms of peptic ulceration. The constitution of Gaviscon preparations varies according to dosage forms. Gaviscon tablets contain alginic acid, dried aluminium hydroxide, magnesium trisilicate and sodium bicarbonate, whereas Gaviscon liquid contains sodium alginate, sodium bicarbonate and calcium carbonate.

A11   D

Famvir is a proprietary preparation of famciclovir (used for the treatment of herpes virus infections).

A12 C

Sporanox is a proprietary preparation of itraconazole (triazole antifungal).

A13 E

Lamisil is a proprietary preparation of terbinafine (antifungal).

A14 E

Amphotericin is active against most fungi and yeasts. It can be used for intestinal candidiasis.

A15 C

Both levofloxacin and ciprofloxacin are quinolones. Levofloxacin has greater activity against pneumococci than ciprofloxacin.

A16 C

Tavanic is a proprietary preparation of levofloxacin.

A17 A

Nalidixic acid is a quinolone that is indicated only for urinary tract infections.

A18 A

Atenolol is a beta-adrenoceptor blocker that, when administered during pregnancy, may cause intrauterine growth restriction, neonatal hypoglycaemia and bradycardia.

A19 D

Carbamazepine is an anti-epileptic drug that, when administered during the first trimester of pregnancy, increases the risk of teratogenesis, including an increased risk of neural tube defects. To counteract the risk of neural tube defects, adequate folate supplements are advised before and during pregnancy. Administration of carbamazepine during the third trimester may cause vitamin K deficiency and increase the risk of neonatal bleeding.

A20 C

Imipramine is a tricyclic antidepressant that, when administered during the third trimester, may cause tachycardia, irritability and muscle spasms in the neonate.

A21 B

The maximum daily dose for diclofenac, a non-steroidal anti-inflammatory drug, is 150 mg.

A22 C

The maximum daily dose for sildenafil, a phosphodiesterase type-5 inhibitor, is 100 mg.

A23 E

The maximum daily dose for sumatriptan, a $5HT_1$-agonist, is 300 mg.

A24 D

Chlorpromazine is an antipsychotic drug, specifically a phenothiazine derivative, that is characterised by pronounced sedative effects. Cautionary labels recommended are to avoid exposure of skin to direct sunlight or sun lamps and a warning that it may cause drowsiness and, if affected, not to drive or operate machinery and to avoid alcoholic drinks.

A25 E

Dapsone is an anti-leprotic drug. It is also used in malaria prophylaxis and in dermatitis herpetiformis. The cautionary label 'Do not stop taking this medicine except on your doctor's advice' is recommended. This label is recommended for use on preparations that contain a drug which has to be taken over long periods without the patient perceiving any benefit, or for a drug where withdrawal is likely to present a particular hazard. In the management of leprosy, dapsone may be used in combination with other drugs and treatment is usually for a few months. Withdrawal of dapsone therapy in skin conditions may be associated with sudden flare-ups.

A26 C

Warfarin is an oral anticoagulant. The cautionary label 'Follow the printed instructions you have been given with this medicine' is recommended. An appropriate treatment card should be given to the patient where advice on anticoagulant therapy, necessity of monitoring and precautions are presented.

A27 E

Alupent, which contains orciprenaline, an adrenoceptor agonist, is available as a syrup.

A28 C

Atrovent, which contains ipratropium, an antimuscarinic bronchodilator, is available as an aerosol for inhalation, as a nebuliser solution, and as dry powder for inhalation.

A29   A

AeroChamber is a proprietary name for a spacer device. It is a large spacer with a one-way valve. Spacer devices eliminate the disadvantage associated with metered-dose inhalers, where drug administration may be compromised due to lack of coordination between actuation of the inhaler and inhalation.

A30   D

Beconase, which contains beclometasone, a corticosteroid, is available as a nasal spray.

A31   C

Klaricid, which contains clarithromycin, a macrolide antibacterial agent, is available as yellow tablets in 250 mg and 500 mg strengths.

A32   A

Diovan, which contains valsartan, an angiotensin-II receptor antagonist, is available as yellow tablets 40 mg.

A33   B

Warfarin, an oral anticoagulant, is available as brown tablets at 1 mg strength. Warfarin is also available as tablets in other colours in the 0.5 mg, 3 mg and 5 mg strengths.

A34   E

Zomig, which contains zolmitriptan, a $5HT_1$-agonist, is available as yellow tablets of 2.5 mg.

A35   B

Cisplatin is a platinum compound that is used alone or in combination therapy for the treatment of testicular, lung, cervical, bladder, head and neck and ovarian cancer. It is administered intravenously and is available as powder for injection. The powder formulation should be reconstituted with water for injections to produce a 1 mg/mL solution. Subsequently it is diluted into 2 L sodium chloride 0.9% or sodium chloride and glucose solution. The infusion is given over 6–8 h.

A36   D

Ceftazidime is a 'third-generation' cephalosporin antibacterial agent. It has greater activity than cefuroxime against certain Gram-negative bacteria and less activity against Gram-positive bacteria. Ceftazidime is administered by deep intramuscular injection or intravenous injection or infusion. It is not available as tablets.

A37   B

Both ergotamine and zolmitriptan are indicated for migraine attacks. When ergotamine and zolmitriptan are administered concurrently there is an increased risk of vasospasm. Use of ergotamine should be avoided for 6 h after administration of zolmitriptan, and use of zolmitriptan should be avoided for 24 h after administration of ergotamine. This reaction could be potentially hazardous. When warfarin is administered to a patient receiving a sulphonyl-urea such as gliclazide, this could enhance the hypoglycaemic effect and may also result in changes in the anticoagulant effect. There is no evidence of a potentially hazardous interaction when clindamycin is administered to patients receiving combined oral contraceptives.

A38   B

Griseofulvin and rifampicin are enzyme inducers. They can increase the rate of synthesis of cytochrome P450 enzymes, resulting in enhanced clearance of other drugs. When enzyme inducers are administered to patients receiving warfarin, a decreased effect of warfarin results. However, warfarin itself is not known to be an enzyme inducer.

A39 E

Zyloric contains allopurinol, which requires dose-reduction in patients with liver disease. Natrilix contains indapamide, a thiazide diuretic that should be avoided in severe liver disease. Nizoral contains ketoconazole, an antifungal agent that should be avoided in liver disease.

A40 A

Capsulitis is a disorder affecting the shoulder joint. It may be caused by un-accustomed movement or overuse. The condition is characterised by inflammation of the fibrous tissue surrounding the shoulder joint.

A41 B

Any facial lesion that is accompanied by swollen lymph glands in the neck requires referral as this suggests systemic disease or an infection. A rash that presents as a butterfly distribution over the nose and cheeks requires referral as this could be caused by systemic lupus erythematosus. This is a rare condition that is associated with auto-antibody formation. A butterfly rash covering the nose and cheeks is a very characteristic symptom. A scaly rash with mild erythema affecting the forehead and eyebrows indicates seborrhoeic eczema. This condition can extend to the nose and pinna of ears. Emollient creams and ointments are useful in the management of this condition as they hydrate the skin.

A42 B

Gaviscon liquid and Bisodol Heartburn Relief tablets contain sodium bicarbonate. Gaviscon liquid also contains sodium alginate and calcium carbonate.

Bisodol Heartburn Relief tablets contain alginic acid and magaldrate in addition to the sodium bicarbonate. Maalox Plus tablets contain aluminium hydroxide, magnesium hydroxide and simeticone.

A43   A

The pain and inflammation associated with a bee sting are caused by agents that include histamine, apamin, which is neurotoxic, and the enzyme hyaluronidase, which breaks down the intercellular tissue structure, promoting the penetration of the venom into the human tissues.

A44   B

Colofac (mebeverine) and Spasmonal (alverine) contain an antispasmodic agent, whereas Fybogel (ispaghula husk) presents a bulk-forming laxative. Alverine and mebeverine are direct relaxants of intestinal smooth muscle, which may relieve pain in irritable bowel syndrome.

A45   E

Paradichlorobenzene is an organic compound that is included in products, such as Cerumol drops, which are intended for ear wax removal. The rationale for its inclusion is based on the ability of paradichlorobenzene to penetrate the ear wax plugs. In Cerumol it is available with chlorobutanol and arachis oil.

A46   B

Because of its antiplatelet effect, the administration of aspirin to patients receiving warfarin is associated with a potentiated anticoagulant effect leading to an increased risk of bleeding. Aspirin decreases platelet aggregation by inactivating cyclo-oxygenase, an enzyme involved in the platelet aggregation pathway through the interference with thromboxane A2. Vitamin K is required for the procoagulation activity. Aspirin does not interfere with vitamin K synthesis. However warfarin, which is an oral anticoagulant, acts as a vitamin K antagonist.

A47   D

Male-pattern baldness is also referred to as androgenetic alopecia. It occurs when genetically predisposed hair follicles in the scalp respond to stimulation by circulating androgens.

A48   A

Finasteride is an inhibitor of the enzyme 5α-reductase, which is responsible for the metabolism of testosterone into the androgen dihydrotestosterone. Finasteride is used in benign prostatic hyperplasia and at a lower dose in male-pattern baldness.

A49   A

Diamorphine is an opioid drug, which in many countries is classified as a 'controlled drug', indicating that special prescription and dispensing requirements are necessary. Diamorphine is more lipid soluble than morphine and this allows for effective doses to be injected in smaller volumes. Diamorphine may be administered by mouth, subcutaneously, intramuscularly or by intravenous injection.

A50   A

The three drugs are used in the management of nausea and vomiting caused by palliative cancer treatment, which commonly features cytotoxics and opioid drugs. The three drugs are useful in counteracting nausea and vomiting

induced by opioids and cytotoxic agents. Haloperidol is also used in palliative care to counteract nausea and vomiting attributable to chemical causes
such as hypercalcaemia and renal failure.

A51   D

Bacterial conjunctivitis is an eye disorder characterised by inflammation of the
conjunctiva caused by a bacterial infection. A common microorganism associated with this condition is *Staphylococcus aureus*. The condition does not
necessarily affect both eyes. However, infection can be spread from one eye
to the other. The patient complains of itchiness or grittiness on the surface of
the eye but this is differentiated from pain.

A52   E

Wet skin lesions or weeping lesions may or may not be infected. Referral is
not always warranted. It is recommended to refer when the lesion is presenting purulent discharge, which indicates an infective component. When the
exudate is clear and watery, the patient may be advised to undertake potassium permanganate soaks to cleanse the lesion.

A53   D

Infant formula milk preparations are manufactured to mimic as much as
possible the composition of the mother's milk. Most preparations are based
on cow's milk, and modifications, such as the addition of carbohydrates, are
made to achieve the formula. The fat content of infant formula milk is adjusted
to be similar to mother's milk. Some preparations may substitute cow's milk fat
with vegetable and animal fats that are more easily digested. Infant formula
milk preparations may be presented as ready-to-use preparations or as
powders for reconstitution. Dried milk formulations should be reconstituted
according to the manufacturer's instructions and involve adding water to the
powder formulation.

A54 C

Staphylococcal napkin dermatitis is a condition where a rash develops in the napkin area. A rash that has a pustular appearance, as opposed to a confluent red rash, which is associated with napkin dermatitis, indicates a bacterial infection caused by the *Staphylococcus* species. A patient presenting such symptoms should be referred as antibacterial treatment may be indicated. Candidal napkin dermatitis, where infection of the napkin area with *Candida* species occurs, is associated with oral thrush (candidiasis).

A55 C

Sialolithiasis is a condition characterised by the formation of calculi (salivary stones) in the salivary ducts or salivary glands. This leads to obstruction and hence accumulation of saliva within the gland especially when eating. The patient presents with facial pain and swelling, which may last for a few hours.

A56 A

A history or suspicion of a perforated ear drum requires referral for assessment of the damage and treatment of the condition through systemic drug administration. Discharge may reflect an infective component such as in otitis media and infective dermatitis. Earache generally occurs with otitis media and requires referral for diagnosis.

A57 B

Enquiry whether the symptoms are related to food intake patterns confirms that the origin of discomfort is in the gastrointestinal tract. Vomiting or constipation with indigestion warrant referral because the clinical presentation may indicate obstruction in the gastrointestinal tract.

A58   A

Products containing adsorbents such as kaolin are not recommended for acute diarrhoea. Adsorption may interfere with the absorption of other drugs from the intestine. Oral rehydration therapy should be considered to be the first-line treatment in acute diarrhoea. Kaolin and Morphine Mixture is an oral suspension that contains 4% chloroform and morphine tincture. Absorption of morphine after oral administration of Kaolin and Morphine may be reduced because it may become adsorbed to the kaolin.

A59   C

Meggezones pastilles contain menthol. They provide a soothing effect for sore throats through the promotion of saliva secretion. The preparation contains glucose as excipients and therefore should not be recommended to diabetic patients.

A60   A

In migraine gastric motility is reduced and this may compromise drug absorption. Soluble oral drug formulations are preferred to solid oral dosage forms because absorption is faster. Analgesics should be taken at the first sign of an attack. Syndol contains paracetamol (non-opioid drug), caffeine, codeine (opioid drug) and doxylamine (antihistamine). Syndol presents a compound analgesic that also contains caffeine, which is a weak stimulant claimed to enhance the analgesic effect, and a sedating antihistamine that confers anti-emetic activity.

A61   B

Hydroxychloroquine and gold are examples of disease-modifying antirheumatic drugs that can be used in the management of rheumatoid arthritis. Hydroxychloroquine is better tolerated than gold. Gold is associated with severe skin reactions and blood disorders, which could be sudden and fatal.

A62   B

Porphyrias are a group of rare disorders that are characterised by a disturbed metabolism of porphyrin, which contributes to the formation of the iron-containing complex, haem. Attacks may be precipitated by drug administration. Progestogens are porphyrinogenic and should be avoided in patients with porphyria.

A63   B

Goserelin is a gonadorelin analogue that can be used in prostate cancer. During the initial weeks of treatment with gonadorelin analogues, increased production of testosterone may result in the progression of prostate cancer (tumour 'flare'). This stage may present with increased bone pain, back pain caused by spinal cord compression, and ureteric obstruction.

A64   D

Tacrolimus and ciclosporin are immunosuppressants. Tacrolimus is a fungal macrolide and has a different chemical structure to ciclosporin. However, it has a similar mode of action.

Tacrolimus

Ciclosporin

A65   C

Imipramine is a tricylic antidepressant and, as with all types of antidepressants, hyponatraemia may occur in older people. This is possibly due to inappropriate secretion of antidiuretic hormone.

A66   E

Inflammation of the larynx (laryngitis) is usually due to a bacterial or viral infection and is a very common condition after a common cold. When the cause of laryngitis is a bacterial infection, an antibacterial agent may be appropriate. Atropine is an antimuscarinic drug that can be used in the symptomatic relief of gastrointestinal disorders characterised by smooth muscle spasm, in mydriasis and cycloplegia, for the reversal of bradycardia, and in cardiopulmonary resuscitation.

A67   A

Lidocaine is indicated for ventricular arrhythmias, especially after myocardial infarction, because it suppresses ventricular tachycardia and reduces the risk of ventricular fibrillation.

A68   A

In moderate kidney damage, the dose of atenolol should be reduced. Atenolol is a highly water-soluble drug that is excreted by the kidneys. Hence it may accumulate in the body to a greater extent than propranolol, which is predominantly excreted by the liver.

A69   C

Filgrastim is indicated for the reduction in duration of neutropenia as a result of cytotoxic chemotherapy. Filgrastim is a recombinant human granulocyte-colony stimulating factor (G-CSF).

A70   E

When drugs are administered to breast-feeding mothers, the concentration of some drugs in milk may exceed the concentration in maternal plasma. Therapeutic doses in the mother may result in toxic doses in the milk. Toxicity in the infant depends on the drug and on the amount of drug in the milk.

A71   C

Pemphigus is a skin condition characterised by severe and chronic blistering, which is attributed to an autoimmune reaction. Oral corticosteroids are the first-line treatment. Immunosuppressants are considered either when optimum management is not achieved with oral corticosteroids or when corticosteroids are not tolerated or the dose has to be decreased.

A72   D

Ear pain during air travel when the aircraft is descending occurs when the eustachian tube, which normally equalises the pressure, is blocked and pressure inside the middle ear is less than on the outside (barotrauma). The tympanic membrane is sucked and may rupture. Nasal decongestants may be used to prevent eustachian tube blockage hence preventing barotrauma.

A73   C

Stelazine contains trifluoperazine, a phenothiazine. It may cause pancytopenia, which includes agranulocytosis. Agranulocytosis is a condition resulting in a marked decrease in the number of granulocytes.

A74   C

Tinnitus is an adverse effect of furosemide, especially when it is administered in large parenteral doses, as a rapid administration and in renal impairment. Not all diuretics are associated with tinnitus.

A75   B

Increased serotonergic effects have been reported when St John's wort is given with selective serotonin re-uptake inhibitors (SSRIs). Concomitant use should be avoided. Sertraline is an SSRI. St John's wort is a herbal remedy that can be used for mild depression.

A76   E

Co-codamol preparations, which may be sold to the public as over-the-counter medicines, contain codeine 8 mg. Co-codamol is a combination of codeine (opioid drug) and paracetamol.

A77   C

Varicella (chickenpox) is an infection caused by the varicella zoster virus, which in the acute phase is highly contagious. It is transmitted via airborne droplets or by contact with active lesions. Varicella zoster immunoglobulin is available for prophylaxis for individuals who are at increased risk of severe varicella or who have significant exposure to chickenpox or herpes zoster.

A78   D

Graduated compression hosiery is in some cases recommended during pregnancy against the varicosis that may result. Compression with graduated hosiery allows haemostasis to occur and therefore reduces oedema and swelling.

A79   D

Nocturnal enuresis is persistent involuntary urination during sleep and it is a common condition in young children. Drug treatment is not appropriate in children under 5 years of age and it is usually not needed in those under 7 years. Psychotherapy and enuresis alarms may be used. Enuresis alarms should be first-line treatment for well-motivated children aged over 7 years because their use may achieve a more sustained reduction of enuresis than the use of drugs. Tricyclic antidepressants such as amitriptyline, imipramine and less often, nortriptyline may be used in nocturnal enuresis. However, relapse is common after drug withdrawal.

A80   D

Betahistine is an analogue of histamine and is indicated for vertigo, tinnitus and hearing loss associated with Ménière's disease. Side-effects of betahistine include gastrointestinal disturbances, headache, rashes and pruritus.

A81 A

Premarin is an example of a product that presents hormone replacement therapy and contains conjugated oestrogens 625 µg.

A82 E

Premarin is also available as tablets of 1.25 mg conjugated oestrogens and as a vaginal cream, which contains 625 µg/g conjugated oestrogens.

A83 C

Premarin is not indicated in women with intact uterus because it does not present cyclical or continuous administration of progestogen. In women with intact uterus, the administration of progestogen for at least 12 days per month reduces the risk of endometrial cancer. Hormone replacement therapy (HRT) is an option for the prophylaxis of osteoporosis and Premarin may be used for this purpose. However, guidelines in a number of countries advise that HRT should not be considered as first-line therapy for the long-term prevention of osteoporosis in women over 50 years of age. Premarin is marketed by Wyeth.

A84 B

Progynova is another product that presents an oestrogen component only and therefore is indicated in women without intact uterus. It contains estradiol valerate. Nuvelle, Trisequens and Femoston are examples of products containing estradiol with progestogen, whereas Prempak-C is an example of a product that contains conjugated oestrogens with progestogen.

A85 D

Patient should take one Premarin tablet daily and start a new pack once the 28-day pack has finished. The therapy is continuous and there is no 7-day break. Patient should be advised to maintain regular visits to a general practitioner every 12 months but should be advised to seek advice from the pharmacist or the general practitioner should any symptoms that warrant withdrawal of the HRT occur. Such symptoms include sudden, severe chest pain, sudden breathlessness or cough with blood-stained sputum, unexplained severe pain in the calf of one leg, severe stomach pain, serious neurological effects including unusually severe, prolonged headache and blood pressure above systolic 160 mmHg and diastolic 100 mmHg.

A86 C

Fosamax contains alendronic acid, a biphosphonate that is adsorbed onto hydroxyapatite crystals in the bone resulting in a deceleration in the rate of growth and dissolution of the bone. Use of alendronic acid therefore results in a decreased rate of bone turnover. Alendronic acid may cause oesophageal reactions and patients should be advised to seek advice if they develop symptoms of oesophageal irritation such as dysphagia.

A87 D

Fosamax Once Weekly is available as a pack containing four tablets of 70 mg strength at a price of £22.80. At this dosage regimen, weekly treatment costs about £6. Fosamax tablets are available in 5 mg, 10 mg and 70 mg strengths. The patient has been prescribed one 70 mg tablet once a week.

A88 B

Combivent contains ipratropium (antimuscarinic bronchodilator) and salbutamol (selective beta$_2$ agonist).

A89 C

Combivent is available as an aerosol inhalation and as a nebuliser solution.

A90 B

Ventolin contains salbutamol and Atrovent contains ipratropium. The two products can be used together to replace the combination product Combivent. Becotide contains beclometasone (corticosteroid).

A91 A

Depo-Medrone consists of methylprednisolone (corticosteroid), which is used for the suppression of inflammatory and allergic disorders and in rheumatic disease.

A92 D

Depo-Medrone is presented as an aqueous suspension that can be administered either by deep intramuscular injection into the gluteal muscle or by intra-articular or intrasynovial injection for rheumatic disease. Administration can be repeated after 2–3 weeks or, for rheumatic disease, at intervals of 7–35 days. Corticosteroids, including methylprednisolone, can be used in the management of raised intracranial pressure or in cerebral oedema resulting from malignancy.

A93 B

Persantin Retard contains dipyridamole which, like aspirin, is an antiplatelet drug.

A94 A

Side-effects of dipyridamole include gastrointestinal effects, worsening of symptoms of coronary heart disease and hot flushes.

A95 D

The original pack of Persantin Retard contains a dessicant that protects the modified-release capsules.

A96 B

The patient should be advised to take one capsule of Persantin Retard twice daily with food and to take one tablet of aspirin daily. Persantin Retard capsules are unstable in humid conditions, so the patient should be advised to open one pack and to use the capsules before opening another pack. If any capsules remain 6 weeks after opening a pack, they should be discarded.

A97 A

Forceval is a multivitamin preparation, which is available as adult and paediatric formulations (Forceval Junior capsules). Vivioptal is also a multivitamin preparation. It is presented for children over 12 years of age and for adults. Maxepa consists of a fish-oil preparation rich in omega-3-marine triglycerides, En-De-Kay presents a fluoride supplement whereas Calcium-Sandoz contains calcium salts.

A98 C

Actifed Chesty Coughs syrup contains guaifenesin (expectorant), pseudo-ephedrine (decongestant) and triprolidine (antihistamine). Benylin with Codeine syrup contains codeine (antitussive), diphenhydramine (antihistamine) and menthol. Alupent syrup contains orciprenaline, an adrenoceptor agonist indicated for reversible airways obstruction. Vicks Medinite syrup contains dextromethorphan (antitussive), doxylamine (antihistamine), ephedrine (decongestant) and paracetamol (analgesic and anti-pyretic). Vicks Medinite is not recommended for children under 10 years of age. Neoclarityn syrup contains desloratidine, a non-sedating antihistamine.

A99   E

Ibutop gel contains ibuprofen. Brufen contains ibuprofen but the dosage forms available are tablets, syrup and effervescent granules. Voltarol (diclofenac) and Oruvail (ketoprofen) present other non-steroidal anti-inflammatory drugs in the form of gels. Dubam products contain rubefacients.

A100   A

Canesten is presented as a vaginal cream, which contains clotrimazole, an imidazole antifungal agent that is indicated in vaginal candidiasis. Ortho-Gynest is presented as an intravaginal cream that contains estriol and which is indicated as a topical hormone replacement therapy. Eurax contains crotamiton, an anti-pruritic, Bactroban contains mupirocin, an antibacterial agent, and Dermovate contains clobetasol, a corticosteroid.

Test 2

Questions

Questions 1–10

Directions: Each of the questions or incomplete statements is followed by five suggested answers. Select the best answer in each case.

Q1   All the following products are selective inhibitors of cyclo-oxygenase-2 EXCEPT:

A   ☐   Celebrex
B   ☐   Arcoxia
C   ☐   Mobic
D   ☐   Feldene
E   ☐   Prexige

Q2   What is an appropriate therapeutic alternative for Pulmicort?

A   ☐   Zaditen
B   ☐   Becotide
C   ☐   Intal
D   ☐   Atrovent
E   ☐   Serevent

Q3   Raynaud's phenomenon:

A   ☐   is characterised by vasodilation
B   ☐   causes hot, red feet
C   ☐   starts as white patches of skin
D   ☐   is caused by a bacterial infection
E   ☐   may require vasodilator treatment

Q4   Leflunomide:

A   ☐   its therapeutic effect starts after 4–6 weeks
B   ☐   is given as an initial dose of 7.5 mg
C   ☐   is administered once a week
D   ☐   is available only for parenteral administration
E   ☐   no washout procedures are required when changing to
          another product

Q5   Zanamivir:

A   ☐   reduces replication of influenza A and B viruses
B   ☐   reduces duration of influenza symptoms by 3 days
C   ☐   is licensed for prophylaxis of influenza
D   ☐   is available as capsules
E   ☐   is licensed for use within 72 h of the first symptoms

Q6   Diabetic retinopathy:

A   ☐   is reversible changes in the lens shape
B   ☐   indicates long-standing uncontrolled diabetes
C   ☐   presents with impaired drainage of the aqueous humour
D   ☐   is an example of corneal injury
E   ☐   is characterised by proteolytic enzymes affecting the lens

Q7   Metolazone:

A   ☐   profound diuresis may occur
B   ☐   is a loop diuretic
C   ☐   is marketed as Natrilix
D   ☐   maximum daily dose is 20 mg
E   ☐   antagonises aldosterone

Q8   All the following products contain codeine EXCEPT:

A   ☐ Syndol
B   ☐ Solpadeine Max
C   ☐ Migraleve
D   ☐ Uniflu
E   ☐ Panadol Extra

Q9   A significant clinical interaction may occur if St John's wort is administered concomitantly with:

A   ☐ gliclazide
B   ☐ simvastatin
C   ☐ sertraline
D   ☐ amoxicillin
E   ☐ salbutamol

Q10   Basal cell carcinoma:

A   ☐ forms metastases rapidly
B   ☐ arises from a mole
C   ☐ may occur in scar tissue
D   ☐ general malaise is the presenting symptom
E   ☐ is associated with poor prognosis

Questions 11–34

Directions: Each group of questions below consists of five lettered headings followed by a list of numbered questions. For each numbered question select the one heading that is most closely related to it. Each heading may be used once, more than once or not at all.

Questions 11–13 concern the following drugs:

A ☐ losartan
B ☐ valsartan
C ☐ candesartan
D ☐ telmisartan
E ☐ lisinopril

Select, from A to E, which one of the above corresponds to the brand name:

Q11 Micardis

Q12 Cozaar

Q13 Diovan

Questions 14–17 concern the following drugs:

A ☐ tramadol
B ☐ dihydrocodeine
C ☐ dextropropoxyphene
D ☐ remifentanil
E ☐ diamorphine

Select, from A to E, which one of the above:

Q14 has fewer of the typical opioid side-effects

Q15 is preferred for use during intra-operative analgesia

Q16 enhances serotonergic and adrenergic pathways

Q17 requires smaller volumes for an equivalent effective dose of morphine

Questions 18–20 concern the following drugs:

A ☐ alfuzosin
B ☐ dinoprostone
C ☐ tadalafil
D ☐ indometacin
E ☐ ritodrine

Select, from A to E, which one of the above:

Q18 may cause drowsiness

Q19 may cause hypokalaemia

Q20 may cause severe uterine contractions

Questions 21–23 concern the following dosage regimens:

A ☐ 5 mg at night
B ☐ 20 mg in the morning
C ☐ 400 µg twice daily
D ☐ 150 mg twice daily
E ☐ 30 mg at night

Select, from A to E, which one of the above corresponds to the following products:

Q21 Dulco-lax tablets

Q22 Zantac tablets

Q23 Pariet tablets

Questions 24–26 concern the following products:

A ☐ Proctosedyl suppositories
B ☐ rifampicin tablets
C ☐ Slow-K tablets
D ☐ isoniazid tablets
E ☐ glycerin suppositories

Select, from A to E, which one of the above corresponds to the following advice:

Q24 swallow whole with fluid during meals

Q25 store between 2°C and 8°C

Q26 advise patient to avoid soft contact lens wear

Questions 27–30 concern the following products:

A ☐ Gaviscon Advance suspension
B ☐ Dentinox drops
C ☐ Eno salts
D ☐ Actonorm gel
E ☐ Rennie tablets

Select, from A to E, which of the above:

Q27 contains sodium bicarbonate

Q28 is suitable for a patient with symptoms of mild gastro-oesophageal reflux disease

Q29 contains calcium salts

Q30 is a preparation that contains simeticone only as active ingredient

Questions 31–34 concern the following tablet descriptions:

A   ☐ greyish-red 25 mg
B   ☐ m/r pink 10 mg
C   ☐ m/r grey-red 75 mg
D   ☐ orange scored 100 mg
E   ☐ white scored 5 mg

Select, from A to E, which one of the above corresponds to the following proprietary preparation:

Q31   Adalat

Q32   Tenormin

Q33   Anafranil

Q34   Ludiomil

Questions 35–60

Directions: For each of the questions below, ONE or MORE of the responses is (are) correct. Decide which of the responses is (are) correct. Then choose:

A   ☐ if 1, 2 and 3 are correct
B   ☐ if 1 and 2 only are correct
C   ☐ if 2 and 3 only are correct
D   ☐ if 1 only is correct
E   ☐ if 3 only is correct

Directions summarised				
A	B	C	D	E
1, 2, 3	1, 2 only	2, 3 only	1 only	3 only

Q35 According to good practice, when dispensing a medication the pharmacist is required to:

1 ❏ provide written instructions
2 ❏ provide verbal advice
3 ❏ ask whether the patient has any problems with the medication

Q36 When a patient presents with symptoms of a musculoskeletal disorder in the neck and arms, which of the following points should be given priority by the pharmacist when assessing the symptoms?

1 ❏ stiffness and numbness
2 ❏ sustained injury
3 ❏ itchiness

Q37 In a community pharmacy, the managing pharmacist should ensure that the dispensing equipment:

1 ❏ is stored in a clean place
2 ❏ is cleaned after use
3 ❏ is securely locked and accessible only to pharmacists

Q38 A female patient presents with uncomplicated symptoms of painful, frequent and urgent urination. When recommending management of the condition, the pharmacist should prioritise:

1 ❏ explaining to the patient about personal hygiene
2 ❏ recommending medications that alkalinise the urine
3 ❏ advising the patient to drink large volumes of fluid

Q39 Which of the following agents is (are) used in fungating growth in palliative care?

1 ❏ metronidazole
2 ❏ amoxicillin
3 ❏ nitrofurantoin

Q40 Paracetamol overdose:

1   ☐ occurs with the ingestion within 24 h of 4 g
2   ☐ early features are hyperventilation and sweating
3   ☐ liver damage is maximal 3–4 days after ingestion

Q41 Which of the following drugs require a dose-reduction in patients with severe renal impairment?

1   ☐ cefaclor
2   ☐ amoxicillin
3   ☐ insulin

Q42 Follitropin alfa:

1   ☐ may be administered by subcutaneous injection
2   ☐ is used in the treatment of infertility in women
3   ☐ infertility caused by thyroid disorders should be ruled out before administration

Q43 Potentially hazardous interactions could occur between:

1   ☐ memantine and Night Nurse
2   ☐ tacrolimus and grapefruit juice
3   ☐ carbamazepine and co-proxamol

Q44 Remicade:

1   ☐ inhibits activity of tumour necrosis factor
2   ☐ is used in rheumatoid arthritis when the patient has not responded to other disease-modifying antirheumatic drugs
3   ☐ the patient should be instructed to seek advice if symptoms suggestive of tuberculosis occur

Q45 Varicella-zoster vaccine:

1 ☐ is a live attenuated vaccine
2 ☐ is indicated for routine immunisation in children
3 ☐ is available in two strengths

Q46 Liver function should be monitored when treatment is started with which of the following drugs?

1 ☐ rosiglitazone
2 ☐ carvedilol
3 ☐ insulin

Q47 Cough preparations that can be used in a patient with hyperthyroidism complaining of a chesty cough include:

1 ☐ Mucodyne
2 ☐ Actifed Chesty Coughs
3 ☐ Day Nurse

Q48 Locabiotal:

1 ☐ is an anti-infective preparation
2 ☐ may be administered nasally or in the oral cavity
3 ☐ is indicated for first-line treatment of bacterial sinusitis

Q49 Which of the following drugs should be avoided with statins?

1 ☐ gemfibrozil
2 ☐ digoxin
3 ☐ co-amoxiclav

Q50 Propofol:

1 ☐ is administered by inhalation
2 ☐ may be used for the induction of anaesthesia in paediatric patients
3 ☐ is associated with minimal hangover effects

Q51 Pyridoxine:

1 ☐ deficiency may occur during isoniazid therapy
2 ☐ may be used daily for the management of premenstrual syndrome
3 ☐ is a precursor of prostaglandin E1

Q52 Effective product(s) for the prophylaxis of motion sickness that can be taken 30 minutes before travelling is (are):

1 ☐ cetirizine
2 ☐ cinnarizine
3 ☐ hyoscine

Q53 Witch hazel

1 ☐ contains flavonoids and tannins
2 ☐ has astringent and anti-inflammatory properties
3 ☐ is indicated for the management of psoriasis

Q54 Leptospirosis:

1 ☐ is caused by a parasitic microorganism found on dogs
2 ☐ onset is sudden
3 ☐ symptoms are similar to influenza but may include abdominal pain and vomiting

Q55 Venous ulcers:

1 ☐ generally occur on the lower leg
2 ☐ patients should be encouraged to exercise
3 ☐ patients should be advised not to use compression bandages

Q56 Cushing's syndrome:

1 ☐ hypersecretion of hydrocortisone occurs
2 ☐ may be caused by long-term systemic administration of prednisolone at high doses
3 ☐ is characterised by loss of weight

Q57 Juvenile rheumatoid arthritis:

1 ☐ has a poor prognosis
2 ☐ affects predominantly lower limbs
3 ☐ bladder function may be impaired

Q58 Dorzolamide:

1 ☐ may be used in conjunction with timolol
2 ☐ may cause eyelid inflammation and crusting
3 ☐ blood count should be monitored

Q59 Aerodiol:

1 ☐ contains an oestrogen component only
2 ☐ may be used with cyclical progestogen
3 ☐ is presented as a nasal spray

Q60 Imatinib:

1 ☐ may cause nephrotoxicity
2 ☐ is given intravenously
3 ☐ is used in chronic myeloid leukaemia

Questions 61–80

Directions: The following questions consist of a first statement followed by a second statement. Decide whether the first statement is true or false. Decide whether the second statement is true or false. Then choose:

A ☐ if both statements are true and the second statement is a **correct explanation** of the first statement

B ☐ if both statements are true but the second statement **is NOT a correct explanation** of the first statement

C ☐ if the first statement is true but the second statement is false

D ☐ if the first statement is false but the second statement is true

E ☐ if both statements are false

Directions summarised			
	First statement	**Second statement**	
A	True	True	Second statement is a *correct explanation* of the first
B	True	True	Second statement is *NOT a correct explanation* of the first
C	True	False	
D	False	True	
E	False	False	

Q61 No important differences have been found between the major classes of antihypertensive drugs in terms of efficacy. The choice of antihypertensive drugs depends on contraindications.

Q62 Citalopram should not be used in patients under 18 years. An increased risk of suicidal thoughts is associated with SSRIs.

Q63 Sodium blood levels should be monitored in patients taking antidepressants reporting drowsiness and confusion. Hypernatraemia may occur with antidepressants.

Q64 Salmeterol should not be used on a regular basis in patients with mild to moderate asthma. Salmeterol should be used as a single therapy in acute attacks.

Q65 An initial daily dose of orphenadrine hydrochloride is 150 mg. The maximum dose is limited by end-of-dose deterioration.

Q66 Differin gel is a retinoid-like drug. Differin gel is applied once daily at night.

Q67 Measles is an acute infection where the catarrhal stage is the most infectious. The MMR vaccine may be used for prophylaxis of rubella following exposure.

Q68 Tinzaparin may be administered 24 h before surgery. Tinzaparin is administered once daily in the prophylaxis of deep-vein thrombosis after general surgery.

Q69 In the prophylaxis of angina, glyceryl trinitrate patches are applied every 8 h. The patch should be applied to the lateral chest wall on the same site every time.

Q70 Alfacalcidol is the hydroxylated form of vitamin D. It is associated with hypercalcaemia, which is difficult to treat.

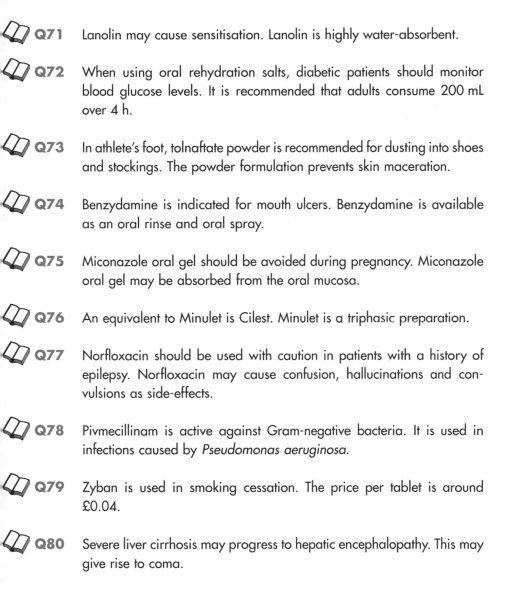

Q71 Lanolin may cause sensitisation. Lanolin is highly water-absorbent.

Q72 When using oral rehydration salts, diabetic patients should monitor blood glucose levels. It is recommended that adults consume 200 mL over 4 h.

Q73 In athlete's foot, tolnaftate powder is recommended for dusting into shoes and stockings. The powder formulation prevents skin maceration.

Q74 Benzydamine is indicated for mouth ulcers. Benzydamine is available as an oral rinse and oral spray.

Q75 Miconazole oral gel should be avoided during pregnancy. Miconazole oral gel may be absorbed from the oral mucosa.

Q76 An equivalent to Minulet is Cilest. Minulet is a triphasic preparation.

Q77 Norfloxacin should be used with caution in patients with a history of epilepsy. Norfloxacin may cause confusion, hallucinations and convulsions as side-effects.

Q78 Pivmecillinam is active against Gram-negative bacteria. It is used in infections caused by *Pseudomonas aeruginosa*.

Q79 Zyban is used in smoking cessation. The price per tablet is around £0.04.

Q80 Severe liver cirrhosis may progress to hepatic encephalopathy. This may give rise to coma.

Questions 81–100

Directions: These questions involve prescriptions or patient requests. Read the prescription or patient request and answer the questions.

Questions 81–85: Use the prescription below:

Patient's name ....
Symbicort turbohaler 200/6
2 puffs bd
Doctor's signature ....

Q81   Each inhalation of Symbicort contains:

A   ☐ budesonide 200 μg and formoterol 6 μg
B   ☐ budesonide 6 μg and formoterol 200 μg
C   ☐ budesonide 160 μg and formoterol 4.5 μg
D   ☐ budesonide 200 mg and formoterol 6 mg
E   ☐ budesonide 160 mg and formoterol 4.5 mg

Q82   Symbicort is presented:

1   ☐ as a pressurised metered-dose inhaler
2   ☐ with a spacer device
3   ☐ as a dry powder inhaler

A   ☐ 1, 2, 3
B   ☐ 1, 2 only
C   ☐ 2, 3 only
D   ☐ 1 only
E   ☐ 3 only

Q83 The patient should be advised to:

1 ☐ use the product twice daily
2 ☐ rinse the mouth with water after inhalation
3 ☐ use the medication on alternate days

A ☐ 1, 2, 3
B ☐ 1, 2 only
C ☐ 2, 3 only
D ☐ 1 only
E ☐ 3 only

Q84 Following long-term use of the product the patient may be predisposed to:

1 ☐ osteoporosis
2 ☐ glaucoma
3 ☐ cataracts

A ☐ 1, 2, 3
B ☐ 1, 2 only
C ☐ 2, 3 only
D ☐ 1 only
E ☐ 3 only

Q85 The patient could monitor management of the condition treated by:

A ☐ nebulisers
B ☐ peak flow meters
C ☐ oxygen flow
D ☐ use of spacers
E ☐ use of respirator solutions

Questions 86–88: Use the prescription below:

Patient's name ....
Warfarin tablets
7.5 mg daily
Doctor's signature ....

Q86 When dispensing the above prescription for a 30-day supply, the amount of tablets that should be dispensed is:

A ☐ 30 tablets of 5 mg and 15 tablets of 1 mg
B ☐ 30 tablets of 5 mg and 30 tablets of 1 mg
C ☐ 30 tablets of 5 mg and 90 tablets of 1 mg
D ☐ 60 tablets of 5 mg and 10 tablets of 1 mg
E ☐ 45 tablets of 5 mg

Q87 The INR for a patient receiving warfarin for treatment of deep-vein thrombosis should be kept at:

A ☐ 1
B ☐ 2
C ☐ 2.5
D ☐ 3
E ☐ 3.5

Q88 If the INR level is elevated, steps that could be taken include:

1 ☐ increase dose of warfarin
2 ☐ stop warfarin
3 ☐ check occurrence of bleeding

A ☐ 1, 2, 3
B ☐ 1, 2 only
C ☐ 2, 3 only
D ☐ 1 only
E ☐ 3 only

Questions 89–91: Use the prescription below:

Patient's name ....
Risperdal 2 mg
bd
Doctor's signature ....

Q89 Risperdal is an antipsychotic that is classified as:

A ☐ butyrophenone
B ☐ thioxanthene
C ☐ atypical
D ☐ substituted benzamide
E ☐ diphenylbutylpiperidine

Q90 The patient is advised:

1 ☐ to take two tablets daily
2 ☐ not to stop medication without medical advice
3 ☐ not to consume caffeine-containing drinks

A ☐ 1, 2, 3
B ☐ 1, 2 only
C ☐ 2, 3 only
D ☐ 1 only
E ☐ 3 only

Q91 Risperidone is to be used with caution in:

1 ☐ epilepsy
2 ☐ Parkinson's disease
3 ☐ schizophrenia

A ☐ 1, 2, 3
B ☐ 1, 2 only
C ☐ 2, 3 only
D ☐ 1 only
E ☐ 3 only

Questions 92–94: Use the prescription below:

Patient's name ....
Duphalac
30 mL tds
Doctor's signature ....

Q92 Duphalac may be indicated for:

1 ❑ bowel cleansing
2 ❑ hepatic encephalopathy
3 ❑ constipation

A ❑ 1, 2, 3
B ❑ 1, 2 only
C ❑ 2, 3 only
D ❑ 1 only
E ❑ 3 only

Q93 Duphalac:

1 ❑ discourages proliferation of ammonia-producing organisms
2 ❑ requires systemic absorption for effectiveness
3 ❑ may cause nausea

A ❑ 1, 2, 3
B ❑ 1, 2 only
C ❑ 2, 3 only
D ❑ 1 only
E ❑ 3 only

Q94 Duphalac:

1 ❑ is available as a solution
2 ❑ needs to be reconstituted before dispensing
3 ❑ should be kept in a refrigerator

A ❑ 1, 2, 3
B ❑ 1, 2 only
C ❑ 2, 3 only
D ❑ 1 only
E ❑ 3 only

Questions 95–96: Use the prescription below:

Patient's name ....

Voltarol Ophtha drops
2 drops bd

Doctor's signature ....

Q95 Voltarol Ophtha is used:

1 ☐ after cataract surgery
2 ☐ for its anti-inflammatory properties
3 ☐ to prevent sepsis

A ☐ 1, 2, 3
B ☐ 1, 2 only
C ☐ 2, 3 only
D ☐ 1 only
E ☐ 3 only

Q96 Voltarol Ophtha Multidose:

1 ☐ should be discarded 4 weeks after opening
2 ☐ a specialist prescription is required
3 ☐ the patient should get UV exposure during treatment

A ☐ 1, 2, 3
B ☐ 1, 2 only
C ☐ 2, 3 only
D ☐ 1 only
E ☐ 3 only

Questions 97–100: For each question read the patient request.

Q97 A patient requests a preparation as a cream for the management of chronic symptoms of haemorrhoids. Which of the following products is the most appropriate?

A ☐ Xyloproct
B ☐ Ultraproct
C ☐ Proctosedyl
D ☐ E45
E ☐ Anusol

Q98 A mother asks for a preparation for head lice. Which of the following agents could be recommended?

A ☐ alcohol
B ☐ phenothrin
C ☐ chlorhexidine
D ☐ cetrimide
E ☐ triclosan

Q99 A patient requests lozenges for sore throat. Which of the following products is the most appropriate?

A ☐ Fungilin
B ☐ Contac
C ☐ Bradosol
D ☐ Nystan
E ☐ Uniflu

Q100 A patient is complaining of ear clogging after air travel. Which of the following products is the most appropriate?

A ☐ Cerumol

B ☐ Sofradex

C ☐ Otosporin

D ☐ Rhinocort Aqua

E ☐ Vicks Sinex

Test 2

Answers

A1   D

Feldene contains piroxicam, which is a non-steroidal anti-inflammatory drug that does not exhibit selectivity for cyclo-oxygenase-2 inhibition. Celebrex (celecoxib), Arcoxia (etoricoxib), Mobic (meloxicam) and Prexige (lumiracoxib) are all selective inhibitors of cyclo-oxygenase-2.

A2   B

Pulmicort contains budesonide, a corticosteroid. Becotide also contains a corticosteroid, beclometasone, which is considered to be equally effective. Zaditen contains ketotifen, which is an antihistamine with an action similar to sodium cromoglicate. Intal contains sodium cromoglicate, which is indicated for prophylaxis of asthma, although in general it is less effective than pro- phylaxis with corticosteroid inhalations. Atrovent contains ipratropium, which is an antimuscarinic bronchodilator that can provide short-term relief in chronic asthma and in chronic obstructive pulmonary disease. Serevent contains salmeterol, which is a long-acting beta$_2$ agonist.

A3   E

Raynaud's phenomenon is characterised by vasospasms of arterioles and arteries in the extremities resulting in blanching, cyanosis and numbness. This is followed by redness and throbbing pain. It is mostly idiopathic in origin and secondary causes include occlusive arterial disease and trauma. It may be triggered by exposure to extreme cold and other factors that may cause vasoconstriction such as smoking. Treatment includes nifedipine because it dilates coronary as well as peripheral arteries. Nifedipine is useful in reducing the frequency and severity of attacks.

A4   A

Leflunomide is a disease-modifying antirheumatic drug that exerts its therapeutic effect 4–6 weeks after initiation of treatment. It is started at 100 mg once daily for 3 days and then a maintenance dose of 10–20 mg once daily is recommended. It is available as tablets at 10 mg, 20 mg or 100 mg strengths. The active metabolite of leflunomide persists for a long period, so washout procedures are required in case of serious adverse effects or before changing to another disease-modifying antirheumatic drug.

A5   A

Zanamivir is an antiviral agent used in influenza because it reduces replication of influenza A and B viruses by inhibiting the viral enzyme neuraminidase. It normally reduces the duration of symptoms by around 1–1.5 days. Zanamivir is not licensed for prophylaxis of influenza. It is indicated for the treatment of influenza and should be started within 48 h of the first symptoms. It is available as a dry powder for inhalation.

A6   B

Diabetic retinopathy is a microvascular complication of diabetes. Optimal blood glucose control in diabetic patients reduces the long-term risks of microvascular damage. Long-standing uncontrolled diabetes leads to microvascular damage including damage to the retina. Diabetic retinopathy may cause permanent opacity of the vitreous humour and eventually blindness may result.

A7   A

Metolazone is a diuretic with actions and uses similar to thiazide diuretics. It interferes with electrolyte reabsorption and is associated with profound diuresis. The maximum daily dose is 80 mg. Natrilix is indapamide.

A8   E

Panadol Extra does not contain codeine. It contains paracetamol and caffeine. Syndol contains paracetamol, caffeine, codeine and doxylamine. Solpadeine Max contains codeine and paracetamol. Migraleve pink tablets contain paracetamol, codeine and buclizine, whereas the yellow tablets contain paracetamol and codeine only. Uniflu tablets contain paracetamol, caffeine, codeine, diphenhydramine and phenylephrine.

A9   C

St John's wort increases serotonergic effects when given with sertraline, a selective serotonin re-uptake inhibitor. It does not show any interactions with sulphonylureas, statins, penicillins and beta-adrenoceptor agonists.

A10   C

Basal cell carcinoma (rodent ulcer) may occur in damaged areas such as areas damaged by ultraviolet light, scar tissue from burns and vaccinations. It arises from the basal layer of the epidermis. It rarely forms metastases. The presenting symptom is a small, firm, pearly, raised nodule that is covered by a thin epidermis. Sometimes the thin epidermis may rupture and the patient presents with ulceration. Treatment comprises removal and this is usually followed by healing of the area.

A11   D

Micardis contains telmisartan, an angiotensin-II receptor antagonist.

A12   A

Cozaar contains losartan, an angiotensin-II receptor antagonist.

A13 B

Diovan contains valsartan, an angiotensin-II receptor antagonist.

A14 A

Tramadol has fewer of the typical opioid side-effects, particularly less respiratory depression, less constipation and a lower potential for addiction.

A15 D

Remifentanil is a short-acting and potent opioid drug, which is preferred for use by injection for intra-operative analgesia compared with pethidine and morphine because it acts within 1–2 minutes. Its short duration of action allows prolonged administration at high dosage without accumulation and with little risk of residual respiratory depression.

A16 A

Tramadol, in addition to its opioid effect, also enhances serotonergic and adrenergic pathways.

A17 E

Diamorphine presents good solubility allowing for smaller volumes to achieve an equivalent effective dose of morphine. This factor is important in patients who are compromised and feeble.

A18 A

Alfuzosin is an alpha-blocker that may cause drowsiness as a side-effect.

A19   E

Ritodrine is a beta$_2$ agonist used as a myometrial relaxant that may cause hypokalaemia as a side-effect.

A20   B

Dinoprostone is a prostaglandin used for induction and augmentation of labour. It may cause uterine hypertonus and severe uterine contractions as side-effects.

A21   A

Dulco-lax tablets contain bisacodyl, a stimulant laxative and are administered in adults as 5–10 mg at night.

A22   D

Zantac tablets contain ranitidine, an H$_2$-receptor antagonist that can be administered as 150 mg twice daily or 300 mg at night.

A23   B

Pariet tablets contain rabeprazole, a proton-pump inhibitor that can be administered as 20 mg daily in the morning.

A24   C

Slow-K tablets contain potassium chloride. They are presented as a modified-release formulation. This requires the patient to be advised to swallow the tablet whole with fluid during meals while sitting or standing to avoid oesophageal or small bowel ulceration caused by the tablet becoming lodged in the gastrointestinal tract.

A25 A

Proctosedyl suppositories present cinchocaine and hydrocortisone in a formulation that the manufacturer recommends that should be stored between 2 and 8°C.

A26 B

Rifampicin causes colouring of body secretions. Because of this side-effect, rifampicin causes discolouration of soft contact lenses and therefore patients should be advised not to wear soft contact lenses during treatment.

A27 C

Eno contains citric acid, sodium bicarbonate and sodium carbonate.

A28 A

Gaviscon Advance suspension includes an alginate that forms a 'raft' on the surface of the stomach contents, which prevents gastro-oesophageal reflux disease. Gaviscon Advance contains sodium alginate and potassium bicarbonate.

A29 E

Rennie contains calcium carbonate and magnesium carbonate.

A30 B

Dentinox colic drops contain simeticone. The product is intended as an anti-foaming agent to be used in infants against gripes, colic and wind pains.

A31 B

Adalat retard tablets are available as 10 mg pink, modified-release tablets.

A32 D

Tenormin tablets are available as orange, scored 100 mg tablets.

A33 C

Anafranil SR is available as grey-red, modified-release 75 mg tablets.

A34 A

Ludiomil is available as greyish-red 25 mg tablets.

A35 A

When dispensing a medication, whether according to a prescription or as a non-prescription medicine, the pharmacist should ask the patient if there are any problems with the medication, such as side-effects or problems with the dosage form. The pharmacist should provide verbal advice and written instructions to ensure proper use of the medication by the patient.

A36 B

Stiffness in the forearm and numbness in the fingers may occur in conditions such as tenosynovitis and carpal tunnel syndrome. Both conditions require referral for further assessment, support structures (splinting may be necessary) and sometimes local steroids. Pain and stiffness with numbness in the neck and arms should be differentiated from symptoms of myocardial infarction. When the patient reports a sustained injury, the pharmacist should assess the extent of the injury to be able to make an informed decision on the line of action to be recommended.

A37 B

In a community pharmacy, the dispensing equipment should be stored in a clean place, properly maintained and cleaned after use. The dispensing equipment should be accessible to personnel who are trained in carrying out the activities pertaining to each equipment.

A38 C

Patient should be advised to drink large volumes of fluid to dilute the bacteria in the bladder. Symptomatic relief of cystitis is achieved by using products that alkalinise the urine, namely sodium citrate and potassium citrate salts. These points should be emphasised to the patient. If counselling time is not restricted, the pharmacist may also discuss points related to personal hygiene. However this issue should not take priority over the other points.

A39 D

Fungating growth may be treated by oral and topical application of metronidazole, which is active against anaerobic and protozoal infections. Metronidazole is available as gel as well as oral formulations.

A40   E

In adults the maximum daily dose of paracetamol should not exceed 4 g. Intake of paracetamol in excess of this dose may cause severe hepatocellular necrosis. Early features of paracetamol overdose are nausea and vomiting that tend to settle within 24 h. Liver damage is maximal 3–4 days after ingestion and this may lead to encephalopathy, haemorrhage and progress to death.

A41   C

Dose-reduction is advised for patients with severe renal impairment receiving amoxicillin and insulin. With amoxicillin, rashes are more common. With insulin, requirements fall and compensatory response to hypoglycaemia is impaired.

A42   A

Follitropin alfa is a recombinant human follicle-stimulating hormone that may be administered by subcutaneous injection. It is used in the treatment of infertility in women who have not responded to clomifene. Infertility caused by thyroid disorders should be ruled out before its administration.

A43   A

Night Nurse contains dextromethorphan, paracetamol and promethazine. Memantine, an N-methyl-D-aspartate (NMDA) receptor antagonist used in dementia, should not be given with products containing dextromethorphan because an increased risk of central nervous system toxicity results. Grapefruit juice should be avoided in patients receiving tacrolimus, an immunosuppressant, as the plasma concentration of tacrolimus is increased. Administration of tacrolimus is associated with a dose-dependent increase in serum creatinine and urea and an incidence of neurotoxicity and nephrotoxicity. When co-proxamol, which consists of paracetamol and dextropropoxyphene, is

administered to patients receiving carbamazepine, the effects of carbamazepine are enhanced.

A44   A

Remicade consists of infliximab, which inhibits the activity of tumour necrosis
factor. It is used for the treatment of active rheumatoid arthritis when the
response to other disease-modifying antirheumatic drugs such as methotrexate
is inadequate. Infliximab has been associated with infections, including
tuberculosis. Patients should be advised to seek advice from the pharmacist or
the prescriber should symptoms suggestive of tuberculosis, such as persistent
cough, fever and weight loss, occur.

A45   D

Varicella-zoster vaccine is a live attenuated vaccine that is not recommended
for routine use in children. It is recommended for individuals with a negative
or uncertain history who come into direct contact with patients. The dosage
regimen for adults involves two doses and for children it normally features one
dose. The vaccine is available in one dosage strength.

A46   B

Liver function should be assessed before starting treatment with rosiglitazone
and carvedilol. Liver dysfunction has been reported with rosiglitazone.
Carvedilol should be avoided in hepatic impairment, and liver function assessment before starting treatment is recommended. Insulin may be used in patients
with hepatic impairment and therefore liver function tests are not required
before treatment.

A47   D

Mucodyne contains carbocisteine, which is a mucolytic that can be used in
patients with hyperthyroidism. Both Actifed Chesty Coughs and Day Nurse

contain sympathomimetics as nasal decongestants. Sympathomimetic agents are contraindicated in patients with hyperthyroidism. Actifed Chesty Coughs contains guaifenesin (expectorant), pseudoephedrine (nasal decongestant) and triprolidine (antihistamine). Day Nurse contains paracetamol (analgesic and antipyretic), pholcodine (antitussive) and pseudoephedrine (nasal decongestant). Day Nurse is not indicated when the presenting complaint is chesty cough.

A48   B

Locabiotal contains fusafungine, which is an anti-infective preparation. It is presented as a metered spray that can be applied nasally or in the oral cavity with different adaptors. It is used for infection and inflammation of upper respiratory tract but is not recommended as a first-line treatment of bacterial sinusitis.

A49   D

When gemfibrozil, a fibrate, is used concomitantly with a statin, there is an increased risk of myopathy. This suggests avoidance of concomitant use. Atorvastatin, a statin, may increase plasma concentration of digoxin. However, this is not a significant interaction that requires avoidance of concomitant use. There are no reported significant interactions between statins and co-amoxiclav.

A50   C

Propofol is an anaesthetic that is administered by intravenous injection or intravenous infusion. It can be used for induction of anaesthesia in paediatric patients over 1 month old. Propofol is widely used because it is associated with rapid recovery with minimal hangover effects.

A51 B

Pyridoxine (vitamin B_6) is used in premenstrual syndrome. Deficiency of pyridoxine is rare but it may occur during treatment with the antituberculous drug, isoniazid.

A52 E

Hyoscine is an antimuscarinic agent that can be used for prophylaxis of motion sickness. Because it has a rapid onset of action it is administered 30 minutes before travelling. Cinnarizine is an antihistamine that is used for the prophylaxis of motion sickness but it has to be administered 2 h before travelling. Cetirizine is a non-sedating antihistamine that is used for symptomatic relief of allergies.

A53 B

Witch hazel contains flavonoids and tannins. It has astringent and anti-inflammatory properties. It is included in ophthalmic preparations.

A54 A

Leptospirosis is caused by an aerobic spirochaete, which is a parasite found on different animals including dogs. The onset is sudden and usually symptoms include fever, chills, myalgia and severe headache. In addition, patient may present with abdominal pain, vomiting, pharyngitis and non-productive cough.

A55 B

Venous ulcers usually involve the superficial veins of the lower leg. Patients should be encouraged to exercise, use graduated compression hosiery or bandages and elevate the legs when in a sitting position.

A56   B

In Cushing's syndrome, the adrenal gland starts overproducing cortisol. This may occur as a result of high doses of corticosteroids such as prednisolone, especially if these are administered on a long-term basis as systemic administration. Characteristic symptoms of Cushing's syndrome include obesity of the trunk and neck, facial rounding (mooning) and reddening, muscle weakness and atrophy, skin atrophy, livid striae, spontaneous bruising and osteoporosis.

A57   D

Juvenile rheumatoid arthritis is rheumatoid arthritis that presents before 16 years of age. The prognosis is poor and it may affect any joint.

A58   B

Dorzolamide is a carbonic anhydrase inhibitor that is administered topically. It may be used as a single-agent therapy or as an adjunct to a topical beta-blocker such as timolol. Side-effects of dorzolamide include ocular burning, stinging and itching, blurred vision, lacrimation, conjunctivitis, eyelid inflammation and crusting.

A59   A

Aerodiol contains estradiol and is used in the management of menopausal symptoms. It can be used with cyclical progestogen in women with intact uterus. It is presented as a nasal spray.

A60 E

Imatinib is a protein-tyrosine kinase inhibitor that is used in chronic myeloid leukaemia. Side-effects include nausea, vomiting, diarrhoea, oedema, abdominal pain, fatigue, myalgia, headache, rash and gynaecomastia. It is administered as an oral preparation in the form of tablets.

A61 B

No important differences have been found between the major classes of antihypertensive drugs in terms of efficacy, side-effects or changes to the quality of life of patients. The choice of an antihypertensive for a specific patient depends on the concurrent conditions (indications) and contraindications. For example, thiazide diuretics are particularly indicated in the elderly and a contraindication for their use is gout.

A62 A

Citalopram is a selective serotonin re-uptake inhibitor (SSRI). SSRIs are associated with suicidal behaviour and this risk is higher in young adults. For this reason SSRIs should not be used in patients under 18 years.

A63 C

Administration of antidepressants has been associated with hyponatraemia. Patients may develop drowsiness, confusion or convulsions.

A64 E

Salmeterol is a long-acting beta$_2$ agonist that can be used regularly in patients with mild or moderate asthma. It can be used in combination with corticosteroid therapy. However, it should not be used in acute asthma attacks.

A65 C

Orphenadrine is an antimuscarinic drug used in the management of parkinsonism. An initial daily dose of 150 mg in divided doses is recommended and the dose can be increased to 400 mg daily. It is not associated with end-of-dose deterioration.

A66 B

Differin gel contains adapalene, which is a retinoid-like drug intended to be applied thinly once daily before retiring.

A67 C

Measles is an acute viral infection that is transmitted by airborne droplet infection. Onset is abrupt and is presented by prodromal symptoms of fever, sneezing, cough, nasal discharge, conjunctivitis, photophobia and myalgia. This stage, referred to as the catarrhal stage, is the most infectious. The live measles, mumps and rubella vaccine (MMR) is intended to eliminate rubella, measles and mumps. MMR vaccine may be used in the control of outbreaks of measles and it can be used within 3 days of exposure to infection. However, MMR vaccine is not suitable for prophylaxis of rubella and mumps following exposure because the antibody response to the mumps and rubella component is too slow for effective prophylaxis.

A68 D

Tinzaparin is a low molecular weight heparin that is administered 2 or 12 h before surgery. When used for prophylaxis of deep-vein thrombosis after general surgery, it is administered once daily for 7 to 10 days.

A69 E

The transdermal patches containing glyceryl trinitrate are changed daily when used for the prophylaxis of angina. The patch should be applied to the lateral chest wall or upper arm. The patch should be applied on a different site every time.

A70 C

Alfacalcidol is the hydroxylated derivative of Vitamin D. Alfacalcidol has a short duration of action and therefore problems associated with hyper-calcaemia due to excessive dosage are short lasting and easy to treat.

A71 B

Lanolin, anhydrous wool fat, is derived from the sebum of sheep and has become less popular because of reports of sensitisation. It is highly water-absorbent and this is the reason why lanolin is used as an emollient.

A72 C

Oral rehydration salts (ORS) contain electrolytes and glucose. In diabetic patients, ORS are recommended in the management of diarrhoea. It is recommended that patients monitor blood glucose levels while receiving oral rehydration salts. Intake of ORS should be adjusted according to fluid loss. In adults around 200 to 400 mL of ORS solution should be consumed after every loose motion or 2–4 litres should be consumed over 4–6 h.

A73 A

Tolnaftate is an antifungal preparation. In the management of athlete's foot, tolnaftate powder may be recommended for dusting into shoes, socks and stockings because it adsorbs moisture thus reducing propagation of the fungus and preventing skin maceration. It may be used either as an adjunct to creams, sprays or ointments in the treatment of an acute phase or as a single agent to prevent recurrence.

A74   B

Benzydamine is an analgesic that is indicated for the management of painful inflammatory conditions of the oropharynx such as mouth ulcers. It is available as an oral rinse and an oral spray.

A75   A

Miconazole is an imidazole antifungal that is available as an oral gel. The gel is to some extent absorbed from the oral mucosa and, because animal studies have shown that miconazole is fetotoxic, miconazole oral gel should be avoided during pregnancy.

A76   E

Minulet and Cilest are examples of combined hormonal contraceptives. Minulet contains gestodene (progestogen) 75 µg and ethinylestradiol (oestrogen) 30 µg. Cilest contains norgestimate 250 µg (progestogen) and ethinylestradiol 35 µg. Both products are monophasic and present a standard-strength preparation of oestrogen. However, Minulet and Cilest vary in the progestogen component presented. Norgestimate is structurally related to levonorgestrel, which is in turn derived from nortestosterone. Gestodene has lower androgenic effects compared with nortestosterone derivatives. It has been associated with an increased risk of venous thromboembolism.

A77   A

Norfloxacin is a quinolone antibacterial agent. Quinolones should be used with caution in patients with a history of epilepsy because they may cause confusion, hallucinations and convulsions as side-effects. They may precipitate convulsions in patients with epilepsy and in those with no previous history of convulsions.

A78   C

Pivmecillinam is the pivaloyloxymethyl ester of mecillinam, an amidinopenicillanic acid derivative. It has significant activity against Gram-negative bacteria including *Escherichia coli* and *Salmonella* species. However it is not active against *Pseudomonas aeruginosa* or enterococci.

A79   C

Zyban contains bupropion, which is used within a smoking cessation programme. Price per tablet is about £0.66.

A80   B

Liver cirrhosis is characterised by destruction of parenchymal cells and changes in the normal structure of the liver. This results in impaired metabolism of ingested substances, including protein. The toxic products resulting from protein metabolism may cause hepatic encephalopathy, which may lead to coma.

A81   C

Symbicort is a metered-dose compound preparation that presents budesonide 160 µg (corticosteroid) and formoterol 4.5 µg (long-acting beta$_2$ agonist) with each inhalation.

A82   E

Symbicort is presented as dry powder for inhalation.

A83   B

The prescription states that the patient should administer two puffs twice daily. Hoarseness and oral candidiasis may occur with inhaled corticosteroids. Occurrence may be reduced by using a spacer and by rinsing the mouth with water after inhalation. Mouth rinsing with water will wash out corticosteroid residues in the mouth that could bring about the onset of oral candidiasis.

A84   A

Long-term use of inhaled corticosteroids may cause a reduction in bone mineral density predisposing patients to osteoporosis and may increase the risk of glaucoma and cataracts.

A85   B

Peak-flow meters are patient-friendly, hand-held devices that estimate air flow from the lungs. They are useful for asthmatic patients to detect deterioration in their condition. Nebulisers are used to administer high doses of a drug as an aerosol for inhalation. Respirator solutions are used with a nebuliser.

A86   E

Warfarin is available as 0.5 mg, 1 mg, 3 mg and 5 mg tablets. The patient could be dispensed 45 tablets of 5 mg tablets and asked to take one and a half tablets daily. This method of administration results in the fewest number of tablets to be taken by the patient.

A87   C

The International Normalised Ratio (INR), which represents the prothrombin time, should be maintained at 2.5 for patients receiving warfarin for the treatment of deep-vein thrombosis. INR is monitored daily or on alternate days during initial treatment and then at longer intervals.

A88   C

The main unwanted effect of warfarin is haemorrhage and the INR level is checked to detect patients who are predisposed to this unwanted effect. When the INR level is elevated this indicates an increase in prothrombin time and therefore a predisposition to bleeding and haemorrhage. Warfarin doses may be omitted or stopped. Occurrence of bleeding should be checked to be able to decide when to restart drug treatment and the dose to be used.

A89   C

Risperdal contains risperidone, which is an atypical antipsychotic. It differs from conventional antipsychotic agents in its pattern of receptor binding.

A90   B

The patient has been prescribed 2 mg twice daily. The 2 mg tablets may be dispensed and the patient is asked to take one tablet twice daily. Withdrawal of antipsychotic drugs may be associated with acute withdrawal syndromes or rapid relapse. The patient should be advised not to stop taking medication without medical advice. Patients with acute and chronic psychoses or mania tend to present problems of compliance with drug therapy. It is important to advise the patient not to stop treatment without medical advice. Risperidone is associated with drowsiness and the patient should be advised that drowsiness may occur, especially if the drug is being used for the first time.

A91   B

Risperidone is used in the management of schizophrenia and mania. It should be used with caution in patients with a history of epilepsy because it may decrease the convulsion threshold. Although the atypical antipsychotics are associated with a lower frequency of extrapyramidal symptoms than the older antipsychotics, they should be used with caution in Parkinson's disease.

A92   C

Duphalac contains lactulose and is an osmotic laxative that is useful in constipation, producing an effect within 48 h. It is also useful in hepatic encephalopathy, which is a neurological syndrome occurring as a result of liver disease. The condition occurs as a result of the toxic substances such as ammonia that accumulate because they are normally metabolised by the liver.

A93   D

Lactulose is a disaccharide that retains water in the bowel, leading to osmotic diarrhoea of low faecal pH. It discourages the proliferation of ammonia-producing microorganisms and this characteristic is an advantage in hepatic encephalopathy.

A94   D

Duphalac is available as a solution ready-for-use.

A95   B

Voltarol Ophtha contains diclofenac and is used during and after cataract surgery. Being a non-steroidal anti-inflammatory drug (NSAID), its anti-inflammatory properties are useful in the post-operative stage. It is also used in other conditions such as accidental trauma and radial keratotomy for its analgesic and anti-inflammatory properties.

A96 D

Products for ophthalmic use should be discarded 4 weeks after opening to prevent contamination. Voltarol Ophtha is a prescription item that does not usually require special prescription from a specialist.

A97 E

Anusol cream contains bismuth oxide, peru balsam and zinc oxide. These are astringents that protect the damaged skin and help relieve local irritation and inflammation. It is a preparation that can be used for mild cases and for long-term use when the symptoms are not associated with an acute phase of inflammation. Xyloproct, Ultraproct and Proctosedyl all contain a corticosteroid component and they are suitable for short-term use during an acute phase. Xyloproct contains aluminium acetate, hydrocortisone, lidocaine and zinc oxide. Ultraproct contains cinchocaine, fluocortolone in the caproate and in the pivalate form. Proctosedyl contains cinchocaine and hydrocortisone. E45 is an emollient that contains light liquid paraffin, white soft paraffin and hypoallergenic hydrous wool fat, which is intended for symptomatic relief of dry skin conditions.

A98 B

Phenothrin-like permethrin is a synthetic pyrethroid that is recommended for head lice. It is rapidly absorbed into the organisms' cuticle causing paralysis. However, resistance may develop. Alcohol is used as a base in lotions presenting anti-lice products. Chlorhexidine, triclosan and cetrimide are antiseptic products.

A99   C

Bradosol lozenges contain benzalkonium, an antiseptic that can be recommended for sore throat. Fungilin lozenges and Nystan pastilles are used in the management of oral and perioral fungal infections. They contain a polyene antifungal agent. Fungilin contains amphotericin and Nystan contains nystatin. Contac is a preparation containing pseudoephedrine, which is available as capsules. Uniflu is a compound preparation used for colds. Uniflu tablets contain caffeine, codeine, diphenhydramine, paracetamol and phenylephrine.

A100 E

Ear clogging after air travel is due to eustachian catarrh and barotrauma. This can be resolved by using oral or topical nasal decongestants that will remove blockage in the postnasal space and the oropharynx where the entrance to the eustachian tube lies. Vicks Sinex contains oxymetazoline, a nasal decongestant. Cerumol is an ear-wax removal product. Sofradex and Otosporin contain a corticosteroid and an anti-infective component intended for ear or ophthalmic use. Sofradex contains dexamethasone (corticosteroid) and framycetin (anti-infective agent) whereas Otosporin contains hydrocortisone (corticosteroid), neomycin and polymyxin B (anti-infective agents). Rhinocort Aqua is a nasal spray containing budesonide, a corticosteroid.

Test 3

Questions

Questions 1–10

Directions: Each of the questions or incomplete statements is followed by five suggested answers. Select the best answer in each case.

Q1 The Medicines and Healthcare Products Regulatory Agency of the United Kingdom announced a phased withdrawal of co-proxamol because:

A ☐ of a high fatality rate due to overdose
B ☐ it contains an unacceptable amount of codeine
C ☐ it was available as a non-prescription medicine
D ☐ it presented manufacturing difficulties
E ☐ it causes addiction

Q2 Arcoxia is preferred to standard NSAIDs:

A ☐ in patients who have cardiac failure
B ☐ in patients who are at high risk of developing gastroduodenal ulcer
C ☐ in dysmenorrhoea
D ☐ when onset of pain relief is required immediately
E ☐ in patients with asthma

Q3 Pericoronitis:

A ☐ is often presented in paediatric patients
B ☐ is caused by dental caries
C ☐ is characterised by bleeding
D ☐ in severe disease metronidazole is required
F ☐ duration of treatment should not exceed 3 days

Q4 The most appropriate preparation that can be used as an alternative to Betnovate cream is:

A ☐ Becotide
B ☐ Cutivate
C ☐ Dermovate
D ☐ Locoid C
E ☐ Eumovate

Q5 All the following adverse effects are associated with the use of memantine EXCEPT:

A ☐ muscle cramps
B ☐ dizziness
C ☐ headache
D ☐ tiredness
E ☐ anxiety

Q6 The maximum daily number of tablets of Largactil 25 mg that can be administered to adults for the management of psychomotor agitation is:

A ☐ 1
B ☐ 2
C ☐ 3
D ☐ 12
E ☐ 30

Q7 Mesalazine

A ☐ should be avoided in patients who are hypersensitive to salicylates
B ☐ is indicated for diverticular disease
C ☐ is available only as tablets
D ☐ is not associated with side-effects related to blood disorders
E ☐ is a prodrug of 5-aminosalicylic acid

Q8   An investigational medicinal product is:

A   ❑ a product intended to induce a specific alteration in the immunological response

B   ❑ a product consisting of a toxin

C   ❑ a product prepared from homeopathic stocks

D   ❑ a pharmaceutical form of an active substance being tested or used in a clinical trial

E   ❑ a product prepared in a pharmacy in accordance with a prescription

Q9   In pharmaceutical manufacturing, the Qualified Person:

A   ❑ ensures that standards of good practice in manufacturing are complied with

B   ❑ establishes the period of validity of the manufacturer's licence

C   ❑ may revoke a manufacturer's licence

D   ❑ ensures that good accounting practices are implemented in the administration department

E   ❑ advises the Licensing Authority on the granting of a manufacturer's licence

Q10   Tetanus vaccine is indicated when a wound is contaminated with:

A   ❑ oil

B   ❑ acid

C   ❑ ethanol

D   ❑ soil

E   ❑ wine

Questions 11–34

Directions: Each group of questions below consists of five lettered headings followed by a list of numbered questions. For each numbered question, select the one heading that is most closely related to it. Each heading may be used once, more than once or not at all.

Questions 11–13 concern the following drugs:

    A   ☐ stavudine

    B   ☐ indinavir

    C   ☐ ritonavir

    D   ☐ atazanavir

    E   ☐ amprenavir

Select, from A to E, which one of the above:

Q11 is a protease inhibitor that may be used to boost the activity of lopinavir

Q12 should be used with caution in patients with a history of peripheral neuropathy

Q13 is not metabolised by cytochrome P450 enzyme systems

Questions 14–17 concern the following products:

    A   ☐ Day Nurse

    B   ☐ Covonia Mentholated Cough Mixture

    C   ☐ Beechams Hot Lemon powder

    D   ☐ Uniflu

    E   ☐ Vicks Medinite

Select, from A to E, which one of the above:

Q14   consists of paracetamol and a sympathomimetic agent only

Q15   may be recommended for patients with hypertension

Q16   contains pholcodine as an antitussive

Q17   preparation includes ascorbic acid

Questions 18–20 concern the following products:

A   ☐ Voltarol
B   ☐ Prempak-C
C   ☐ Yasmin
D   ☐ Cilest
E   ☐ Diflucan

Select, from A to E, which one of the above products is presented as:

Q18   single-capsule pack

Q19   calendar pack

Q20   dispersible tablets

Questions 21–23 concern the following products:

A   ☐ Aredia
B   ☐ Remicade
C   ☐ Meronem
D   ☐ Zinacef
E   ☐ Zofran

Select, from A to E, for which one of the above:

Q21 infusion should be started within 3 h of reconstitution

Q22 is not to be given with infusion fluids containing calcium

Q23 infusion should be carried out over at least 2 h

Questions 24–26 concern the following drugs:

A ☐ carvedilol
B ☐ spironolactone
C ☐ flecainide
D ☐ rabeprazole
E ☐ misoprostol

Select, from A to E, which one of the above is indicated in:

Q24 Zollinger-Ellison syndrome

Q25 nephrotic syndrome

Q26 arrhythmias associated with Wolff-Parkinson-White syndrome

Questions 27–30 concern the following drugs:

A ☐ co-trimoxazole
B ☐ ephedrine
C ☐ alcohol
D ☐ aspirin
E ☐ chloramphenicol

Select, from **A** to **E**, during breast-feeding, which of the above:

Q27   may reduce milk consumption

Q28   may cause bone-marrow toxicity in the infant

Q29   results in a risk of kernicterus in jaundiced infants

Q30   may cause the infant to present with disturbed sleep

Questions 31–34 concern the use of the following products in paediatric patients:

A   ☐   Seroquel
B   ☐   Xyzal
C   ☐   Stemetil
D   ☐   Largactil
E   ☐   Tofranil

Select, from **A** to **E**, which one of the above:

Q31   is not recommended for use in children

Q32   may be used in autism

Q33   may be used for nocturnal enuresis

Q34   may be used in nausea and vomiting

Questions 35–60

Directions: For each of the questions below, ONE or MORE of the responses is (are) correct. Decide which of the responses is (are) correct. Then choose:

A ☐ if 1, 2 and 3 are correct
B ☐ if 1 and 2 only are correct
C ☐ if 2 and 3 only are correct
D ☐ if 1 only is correct
E ☐ if 3 only is correct

Directions summarised				
A	B	C	D	E
1, 2, 3	1, 2 only	2, 3 only	1 only	3 only

Q35 Extrasystoles:

1 ☐ may be associated with rheumatic heart disease
2 ☐ may be asymptomatic
3 ☐ commonly require digoxin

Q36 Factors that predispose infants to a higher risk of sudden infant death syndrome include:

1 ☐ premature birth
2 ☐ electrolyte imbalance
3 ☐ breast-feeding

Q37 In patients with haemophilia:

1 ☐ dried factor VIII fraction prepared from human plasma is indicated
2 ☐ desmopressin injection may be used as an adjunct drug
3 ☐ administration of sertraline requires monitoring for occurrence of bleeding

Q38   Vitiligo:

1   ☐ may occur in association with diabetes mellitus
2   ☐ spreads rapidly to affect the entire skin
3   ☐ topical corticosteroids are the mainstay of treatment

Q39   Mumps:

1   ☐ has an incubation period of about 14 days
2   ☐ is caused by paramyxoviruses
3   ☐ may be associated with encephalitis that could have a sudden onset

Q40   Computed tomography:

1   ☐ is used to investigate any part of the body
2   ☐ involves exposure to X-rays more than an ordinary X-ray examination
3   ☐ can take pictures of the tissues from almost every angle

Q41   Pleural biopsy:

1   ☐ is used to identify tuberculous pleural effusions
2   ☐ pneumothorax may be a complication
3   ☐ involves biopsy of ascites fluid

Q42   Weight loss is classified as a symptom suggestive of serious disease:

1   ☐ when this is unexplained
2   ☐ because it may be caused by carcinoma
3   ☐ and requires referral when occurring with abdominal symptoms

Q43 Medication storage requirements in a pharmacy include:

1 ☐ temperature control for medicines that are temperature labile
2 ☐ separation of storage of medicines from non-pharmaceutical products
3 ☐ locked cabinet for controlled drugs

Q44 The chemical structure for triamcinolone includes:

1 ☐ cyclic acetonides at the 16 and 17 positions of glucocorticoids
2 ☐ fluorination that enhances glucocorticoid activity
3 ☐ 6α substitution to increase mineralocorticoid activity

Q45 Ibuprofen is:

1 ☐ a reversible inhibitor of cyclo-oxygenase
2 ☐ an organic acid
3 ☐ a suppressor of leukotriene formation

Q46 Pseudoephedrine is:

1 ☐ a stereoisomer of ephedrine
2 ☐ a CNS-stimulant
3 ☐ contained in Day Nurse

Q47 Which of the following products are presented as a long-acting depot injection?

1 ☐ risperidone
2 ☐ prochlorperazine
3 ☐ quetiapine

Q48   Feldene Melt tablets:

1   ☐ require reconstitution with potable water
2   ☐ are fast dissolving tablets
3   ☐ are taken after food

Q49   Isoflurane:

1   ☐ is presented as a liquid for injection
2   ☐ causes potentiation of atracurium
3   ☐ increases risk of arrhythmias when given with adrenaline

Q50   Clinical significant drug interactions with atenolol could occur with:

1   ☐ Yasmin
2   ☐ Deltacortril
3   ☐ Cordarone X

Q51   Plaquenil:

1   ☐ is used in the management of active rheumatoid disease of moderate inflammatory activity
2   ☐ requires regular monitoring of visual acuity
3   ☐ side-effects include pulmonary fibrosis

Q52   Drugs that should be avoided in severe liver disease include:

1   ☐ Bezalip
2   ☐ NovoNorm
3   ☐ Septrin

Q53 Co-Diovan:

1 ☐ includes a specific angiotensin-II receptor antagonist
2 ☐ includes a thiazide diuretic
3 ☐ may be used in diabetic nephropathy

Q54 In diabetic neuropathy:

1 ☐ ibuprofen may relieve mild to moderate pain
2 ☐ gabapentin is an effective alternative to a tricyclic antidepressant
3 ☐ metoclopramide is licensed to treat neuropathic pain

Q55 Levitra:

1 ☐ contains vardenafil
2 ☐ onset of action may be delayed when drug is administered with intake of high-fat meal
3 ☐ acts by causing smooth muscle relaxation

Q56 Syndol:

1 ☐ is a compound analgesic preparation
2 ☐ contains a sedating antihistamine
3 ☐ each tablet contains 1 g paracetamol

Q57 Ikorel:

1 ☐ has arterial vasodilating properties
2 ☐ cannot be used with nifedipine
3 ☐ is contraindicated in hypertensive patients

Q58 Plasma concentration of phenytoin is increased by:

1 ☐ amoxicillin
2 ☐ doxycycline
3 ☐ clarithromycin

Q59 Patients should be advised to swallow tablets whole for:

1 ☐ Fosamax
2 ☐ Xatral XL
3 ☐ Natrilix SR

Q60 Problems with the use of crude coal tar in psoriasis include:

1 ☐ harmful to normal skin
2 ☐ smell
3 ☐ contact allergy may occur

Questions 61–80

Directions: The following questions consist of a first statement followed by a second statement. Decide whether the first statement is true or false. Decide whether the second statement is true or false. Then choose:

A ☐ if both statements are true and the second statement is a **correct explanation** of the first statement
B ☐ if both statements are true but the second statement **is NOT a correct explanation** of the first statement
C ☐ if the first statement is true but the second statement is false
D ☐ if the first statement is false but the second statement is true
E ☐ if both statements are false

Directions summarised			
	First statement	**Second statement**	
A	True	True	Second statement is a *correct explanation* of the first
B	True	True	Second statement is *NOT a correct explanation* of the first
C	True	False	
D	False	True	
E	False	False	

Q61 Terbinafine is an allylamine derivative. Terbinafine clears infection more quickly than the imidazole antifungals.

Q62 Coversyl should not be administered with low-dose spironolactone. An increased risk of hyperkalaemia may occur with concomitant use.

Q63 Rebound congestion occurs more quickly with topical administration of ephedrine than with xylometazoline. Xylometazoline is a longer-acting sympathomimetic.

Q64 A disadvantage of suppositories for haemorrhoids is that the active ingredients may bypass the anal areas. Suppositories are preferred for the treatment of haemorrhoids.

Q65 Autoimmune thrombocytopenia purpura may be presented by scattered petechiae, epistaxis and menorrhagia. Prednisolone 1 mg/kg daily is used to achieve an increase in the platelet count.

Q66 Methylphenidate may cause euphoria. Monitoring of growth is not required with methylphenidate.

Q67 A corticosteroid may be recommended with docetaxel treatment. The corticosteroid is used to reduce fluid retention.

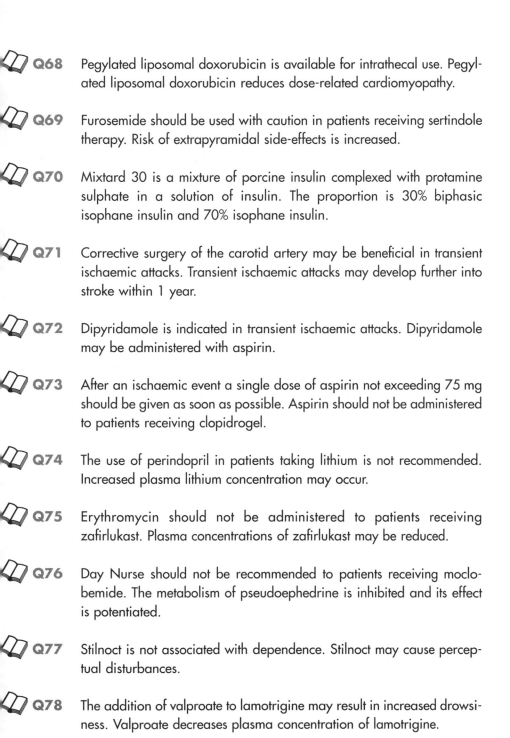

Q68 Pegylated liposomal doxorubicin is available for intrathecal use. Pegylated liposomal doxorubicin reduces dose-related cardiomyopathy.

Q69 Furosemide should be used with caution in patients receiving sertindole therapy. Risk of extrapyramidal side-effects is increased.

Q70 Mixtard 30 is a mixture of porcine insulin complexed with protamine sulphate in a solution of insulin. The proportion is 30% biphasic isophane insulin and 70% isophane insulin.

Q71 Corrective surgery of the carotid artery may be beneficial in transient ischaemic attacks. Transient ischaemic attacks may develop further into stroke within 1 year.

Q72 Dipyridamole is indicated in transient ischaemic attacks. Dipyridamole may be administered with aspirin.

Q73 After an ischaemic event a single dose of aspirin not exceeding 75 mg should be given as soon as possible. Aspirin should not be administered to patients receiving clopidrogel.

Q74 The use of perindopril in patients taking lithium is not recommended. Increased plasma lithium concentration may occur.

Q75 Erythromycin should not be administered to patients receiving zafirlukast. Plasma concentrations of zafirlukast may be reduced.

Q76 Day Nurse should not be recommended to patients receiving moclobemide. The metabolism of pseudoephedrine is inhibited and its effect is potentiated.

Q77 Stilnoct is not associated with dependence. Stilnoct may cause perceptual disturbances.

Q78 The addition of valproate to lamotrigine may result in increased drowsiness. Valproate decreases plasma concentration of lamotrigine.

Q79 In tonic-clonic seizures lamotrigine and sodium valproate are preferred in patients who are on combined oral contraceptives. They are hepatic enzyme inducers.

Q80 Breast-feeding is contraindicated when the mother is receiving an anti-epileptic drug. Anti-epileptic drugs are present in milk in significantly high amounts.

Questions 81–100

Directions: These questions involve prescriptions or patient requests. Read the prescription or patient request and select the best answer in each case.

Questions 81–85: Use the prescription below:

```
┌─────────────────────────────────────────────────────────────┐
│                                                              │
│   Patient's name        ..................................   │
│                                                              │
│   Tavanic 500 mg                                             │
│   bd for 7 days    m 14                                      │
│                                                              │
│                                                              │
│   Doctor's signature    ..................................   │
│                                                              │
└─────────────────────────────────────────────────────────────┘
```

Q81 Tavanic:

1 ☐ contains a quinolone
2 ☐ is active against pneumococci
3 ☐ is a bactericidal product

A   ☐ 1, 2, 3
B   ☐ 1, 2 only
C   ☐ 2, 3 only
D   ☐ 1 only
E   ☐ 3 only

Q82   Tavanic:

1   ☐ is indicated as first-line treatment in uncomplicated lower urinary tract infection
2   ☐ only 250 mg tablets are available
3   ☐ treatment as prescribed in this prescription costs over £30

A   ☐ 1, 2, 3
B   ☐ 1, 2 only
C   ☐ 2, 3 only
D   ☐ 1 only
E   ☐ 3 only

Q83   The patient could be advised:

1   ☐ to avoid excessive exposure to sunlight
2   ☐ that dizziness may occur
3   ☐ to take drug before meals

A   ☐ 1, 2, 3
B   ☐ 1, 2 only
C   ☐ 2, 3 only
D   ☐ 1 only
E   ☐ 3 only

Q84 Tavanic should be avoided in patients who are receiving:

1 ☐ Voltarol
2 ☐ Gaviscon
3 ☐ Tofranil

A ☐ 1, 2, 3
B ☐ 1, 2 only
C ☐ 2, 3 only
D ☐ 1 only
E ☐ 3 only

Q85 A suitable alternative to Tavanic is:

A ☐ Avelox
B ☐ Ciproxin
C ☐ Utinor
D ☐ Fucidin
E ☐ Klaricid

Questions 86–88: Use the prescription below:

Patient's name ....

Daktarin oral gel
5 mL bd

Doctor's signature ....

Q86   Daktarin oral gel:

1   ❑ results in no systemic absorption
2   ❑ requires storage at a temperature between 2 and 8°C
3   ❑ is indicated for treatment of oral candidiasis

A   ❑ 1, 2, 3
B   ❑ 1, 2 only
C   ❑ 2, 3 only
D   ❑ 1 only
E   ❑ 3 only

Q87   Daktarin:

1   ❑ contains miconazole
2   ❑ is available also as powder
3   ❑ is contraindicated in children aged under 5 years

A   ❑ 1, 2, 3
B   ❑ 1, 2 only
C   ❑ 2, 3 only
D   ❑ 1 only
E   ❑ 3 only

Q88   The patient should be advised:

1   ❑ to apply after food
2   ❑ to keep applying product for 2 days after symptoms abate
3   ❑ to apply gel with clean finger and rinse mouth immediately

A   ❑ 1, 2, 3
B   ❑ 1, 2 only
C   ❑ 2, 3 only
D   ❑ 1 only
E   ❑ 3 only

Questions 89–90: Use the prescription below:

Patient's name　　　...

Dexa-Rhinaspray Duo
1 puff tds

Doctor's signature　　...

Q89 Dexa-Rhinaspray Duo consists of:

A　☐　dexamethasone only

B　☐　dexamethasone and an antihistamine

C　☐　dexamethasone and an alpha-adrenoceptor blocker

D　☐　dexamethasone and an alpha-adrenoceptor agonist

E　☐　dexamethasone and a beta-adrenoceptor blocker

Q90 Dexa-Rhinaspray Duo:

1　☐　is not indicated in a child of 4 years

2　☐　nasal bleeding may occur with administration

3　☐　should be stored at 2 to 8°C

A　☐　1, 2, 3

B　☐　1, 2 only

C　☐　2, 3 only

D　☐　1 only

E　☐　3 only

Questions 91–96: Use the prescription below:

Patient's name   ....

Zomig tablets
prn

Doctor's signature   ....

Q91   Zomig:

A   ☐   is a selective antagonist
B   ☐   interacts with the dopaminergic receptors
C   ☐   causes vasoconstriction
D   ☐   is excreted largely by the kidney
E   ☐   presents difficulties in absorption

Q92   The patient should be advised:

1   ☐   to take drug daily
2   ☐   not to exceed intake of four tablets in a day
3   ☐   that drowsiness may occur

A   ☐   1, 2, 3
B   ☐   1, 2 only
C   ☐   2, 3 only
D   ☐   1 only
E   ☐   3 only

Q93 Zomig is contraindicated in:

1 ☐ uncontrolled hypertension
2 ☐ history of transient ischaemic attacks
3 ☐ treatment of acute migraine attacks

A ☐ 1, 2, 3
B ☐ 1, 2 only
C ☐ 2, 3 only
D ☐ 1 only
E ☐ 3 only

Q94 Zomig cannot be prescribed to patients who are taking:

1 ☐ Yasmin
2 ☐ Losec
3 ☐ St John's wort

A ☐ 1, 2, 3
B ☐ 1, 2 only
C ☐ 2, 3 only
D ☐ 1 only
E ☐ 3 only

Q95 Zomig is presented:

1 ☐ as tablets available in a monthly pack
2 ☐ with a cost per tablet of £0.20
3 ☐ by AstraZeneca

A ☐ 1, 2, 3
B ☐ 1, 2 only
C ☐ 2, 3 only
D ☐ 1 only
E ☐ 3 only

Q96   An appropriate substitute to Zomig is:

A   ❑   Migril
B   ❑   Migraleve
C   ❑   Sanomigran
D   ❑   Imigran
E   ❑   Syndol

Questions 97–100: Read the patient request.

A 45-year-old lady presents complaining of heartburn. She states that she gets a sore feeling in her throat area together with stomach problems. She has been having the symptoms for a few days during the past 10 days. There are no symptoms suggestive of serious disease.

For the following products, place your order of preference starting with 4 for the product that should be recommended as first choice and ending with 1 for the product that should be recommended as a last choice.

Q97   Gaviscon liquid

Q98   Phillips' Milk of Magnesia

Q99   Sodium bicarbonate

Q100   Maalox

Test 3

Answers

A1   A

Co-proxamol consists of a combination of dextropropoxyphene and paraceta-mol. In the United Kingdom, the Medicines and Healthcare Products Regulatory Agency has announced a phased withdrawal of co-proxamol because of a high fatality rate caused by overdose. It was reported to be a prescription product commonly associated with death. In overdosage, which may be combined with alcohol consumption, respiratory depression and acute heart failure occur because of the dextropropoxyphene component and hepatoxicity occurs due to paracetamol.

A2   B

Arcoxia contains etoricoxib, which is an NSAID, specifically a cyclo-oxygenase-2 inhibitor. Because of recent reports regarding cardiovascular safety of this class of compounds, etoricoxib should be used with caution in patients with a history of cardiac failure. It should be used in preference to standard NSAIDs in patients who are at a particularly high risk of developing gastroduodenal ulceration, perforation or bleeding, such as in patients with a history of peptic ulceration. Worsening of asthma may be related to the use of NSAIDs.

A3   D

Pericoronitis is an infection occurring in the soft tissue covering impacted wisdom teeth. It occurs during the eruption period of these teeth, usually in adults between 18 and 25 years. It is characterised by pain and swelling. Treatment includes metronidazole or amoxicillin for 3 days or until symptoms resolve.

A4   B

Betnovate cream contains the corticosteroid betamethasone and is a potent preparation. Cutivate contains fluticasone and is also a potent corticosteroid preparation. Dermovate contains clobetasol, which is a very potent cortico-steroid. Locoid C contains hydrocortisone butyrate (a potent corticosteroid) and chlorquinaldol (an antimicrobial agent). Eumovate contains clobetasone, a moderately potent corticosteroid. Becotide is a preparation that contains beclometasone, another corticosteroid, and this is presented for inhalation and not for dermatological use.

A5   A

Muscle cramps are not reported with the use of memantine, which is a NMDA-receptor antagonist used to treat Alzheimer's disease. Dizziness, headache, tiredness and, less commonly, anxiety may occur with memantine adminis-tration.

A6   D

Largactil is chlorpromazine, a phenothiazine that may be used at a maximum daily dose of 300 mg for adults in the management of psychomotor agitation. Twelve tablets daily of Largactil 25 mg would be necessary to achieve this dose.

A7   A

Mesalazine (5-aminosalicylic acid) is an aminosalicylate indicated for treat-ment of mild-to-moderate ulcerative colitis and maintenance of remission. It is contraindicated in individuals who are hypersensitive to salicylates. Side-effects include blood disorders, namely agranulocytosis, aplastic anaemia, leucopenia, neutropenia and thrombocytopenia. Pharmaceutical formulations include tablets, enema and suppositories.

A8   D

An investigational medicinal product is a pharmaceutical form of an active substance being tested or used in a clinical trial. Manufacture of investigational medicinal products has to be undertaken at a site with a manufacturer's authorisation for investigational medicinal products (IMP). The testing has to be coordinated by a named sponsor who will be responsible to see that regulations are complied with.

A9   A

In the pharmaceutical industry, the Qualified Person certifies that each batch of the medicinal products has been produced according to the respective marketing authorisation and in compliance with good manufacturing practice standards.

A10   D

Tetanus is caused by the microorganism *Clostridium tetani*. The spores of this microorganism are found in soil and in faeces. Tetanus-prone wounds include wounds contaminated with soil and manure.

A11   C

Both lopinavir and ritonavir are protease inhibitors used in HIV infection. Ritonavir may be used with lopinavir as a pharmacokinetic enhancer, thus boosting the activity of lopinavir.

A12   A

Stavudine is a nucleoside reverse transcriptase inhibitor used in HIV infection. Side-effects of stavudine include peripheral neuropathy that is characterised by persistent numbness, tingling or pain in feet and hands. It should be used with caution in patients with a history of peripheral neuropathy.

A13   A

Stavudine is not metabolised by cytochrome P450 enzyme systems and the importance of this characteristic is that the potential for drug interactions is low. Protease inhibitors are metabolised by cytochrome P450 enzyme systems and therefore they are potentially associated with significant drug interactions.

A14   C

Beechams Hot Lemon powder contains paracetamol (analgesic and antipyretic) and phenylephrine, a sympathomimetic agent that acts as a nasal decongestant.

A15   B

All the products except Covonia Mentholated Cough Mixture contain a sympathomimetic agent used as a nasal decongestant. Systemic administration of sympathomimetic agents should be undertaken with caution in patients with hypertension. Covonia Mentholated Cough Mixture contains liquorice, menthol and squill.

A16   A

Day Nurse liquid contains paracetamol (analgesic and antipyretic), pholcodine (antitussive) and pseudoephedrine (nasal decongestant).

A17   D

The pack of Uniflu is presented with Gregovite C, which includes a tablet that contains vitamin C, ascorbic acid. Uniflu tablets contain caffeine, codeine (antitussive), diphenhydramine (antihistamine), paracetamol (analgesic and antipyretic) and phenylephrine (nasal decongestant).

A18   E

Diflucan contains fluconazole, which is a triazole antifungal agent that is used as a single dose of 150 mg for the management of vaginal candidiasis and candidal balanitis. Diflucan is available as a single-capsule pack.

A19   B

Prempak-C presents a formulation for hormone replacement therapy containing conjugated oestrogens and norgestrel. It is intended for women with an intact uterus and presents cyclical progestogen for the last 12 days of the cycle. The patient has to take one tablet containing conjugated oestrogens daily and a tablet containing norgestrel on days 17 to 28 of each 28-day treatment. Prempak-C presents the two tablets in a calendar pack, so that the patient will be able to take the norgestrel-containing tablets on the appropriate days.

A20   A

Voltarol contains diclofenac (NSAID) and is available for systemic use as dispersible tablets, tablets, injections and suppositories.

A21   B

Remicade contains infliximab and is available as powder for reconstitution for administration as an intravenous infusion. Once reconstituted, infusion should be started within 3 h.

A22   A

Aredia contains disodium pamidronate, a biphosphonate available for intravenous infusion. It should not be administered with infusion fluids containing calcium because this may interfere with administration of disodium pamidronate.

A23 B

Intravenous infusion of Remicade should be carried out over at least 2 h.

A24 D

Zollinger-Ellison syndrome is characterised by increased plasma gastrin concentration and hypersecretion of gastric acid. Rabeprazole is a proton pump inhibitor that is used in the management of this condition.

A25 B

Nephrotic syndrome is characterised by increased glomerular permeability to protein resulting in proteinuria and marked generalised oedema. Spironolactone, a potassium-sparing diuretic is used in the management of oedema due to nephrotic syndrome.

A26 C

Flecainide is a drug used for arrhythmias that can be administered in the management of arrhythmias associated with Wolff-Parkinson-White syndrome.

A27 C

Large amounts of alcohol consumption during breast-feeding may affect the infant and result in reduced milk consumption.

A28 E

It is recommended to avoid using chloramphenicol during breast-feeding. Chloramphenicol is an antibacterial agent. It may cause bone-marrow toxicity in the infant.

A29 A

Co-trimoxazole presents a mixture of trimethoprim and sulfamethoxazole. When administered to breast-feeding mothers there is a small risk of kernicterus in jaundiced infants.

A30 B

Ephedrine is a sympathomimetic agent and when used in breast-feeding mothers, irritability and disturbed sleep in the infant have been reported.

A31 A

Seroquel contains quetiapine, an atypical antipsychotic. It is not recommended for use in children and adolescents.

A32 D

Largactil contains chlorpromazine, which may be used in childhood schizophrenia and in autism.

A33 E

Tofranil contains imipramine, a tricyclic antidepressant that may be used for nocturnal enuresis in children.

A34 C

Stemetil contains prochlorperazine, a phenothiazine drug that may be used in nausea and vomiting in children.

A35 B

Extrasystoles, also referred to as ectopic beats, are cardiac contractions that occur at an earlier stage during the cardiac cycle. Extrasystoles may be associated with rheumatic heart disease, ischaemic heart disease and acute myocardial infarction. Extrasystoles may be asymptomatic. Digoxin is now rarely used for the management of arrhythmias. Anti-arrhythmic drugs are preferred in the management of extrasystoles.

A36 B

Factors that predispose to sudden infant death syndrome are still not very clear. However, premature birth, electrolyte imbalance and bottle-feeding have been associated with a higher risk.

A37 A

Dried factor VIII fraction prepared from human plasma is used in haemophilia as a treatment and for prophylaxis against haemorrhage. Desmopressin, a posterior pituitary hormone is used as an adjunct to factor VIII to boost concentrations of factor VIII. It is administered as an injection. Sertraline is a selective serotonin re-uptake inhibitor and these drugs are associated with a risk of bleeding disorders especially gastrointestinal.

A38 D

Vitiligo is a dermatological condition that presents with lesions devoid of pigment. It occurs in association with conditions such as diabetes mellitus. It spreads gradually and commonly affects face, neck and exposed areas such as hands, elbows, knees, ankles and feet. Management is based on cosmetic camouflage preparations.

A39 A

Mumps is caused by the paramyxoviruses and has an incubation period of 14–18 days. Encephalitis is not so common but when it occurs it could have serious consequences such as convulsions. Encephalitis, which is inflammation of the brain, could have a sudden or insidious onset.

A40 B

Computed tomography (CT) was originally developed for scanning the brain but nowadays it is used to investigate any part of the body for internal injuries and tumours. A CT scanner sends out several X-ray beams from different angles and there is a greater exposure to X-rays than with an ordinary radiograph. Scanning of the tissues is only horizontal, unlike magnetic resonance imaging (MRI), which can take pictures of tissues from almost any angle.

A41 B

Pleural biopsy is a procedure where biopsy of the pleura is undertaken. Pleural fluid and pleural samples are collected. It is carried out to identify tuberculous pleural effusion, pleural effusion of unknown aetiology and malignant pleural effusion. The most common complication is pneumothorax.

A42 A

Weight loss that cannot be explained by the patient, for reasons such as following a diet or increasing exercise schedule, should always be investigated because it is a symptom suggestive of serious disease. When it occurs with abdominal symptoms, it could indicate underlying pathology such as a peptic ulcer. It could also be caused by carcinoma even if there are no other symptoms.

A43 A

It should be ensured that pharmaceutical products in the pharmacy are maintained in good conditions. Temperature control for medicines that are temperature labile should be undertaken. Storage of medicines should be separate from non-pharmaceutical products. For controlled drugs, special provisions may apply, such as keeping them in a locked cabinet.

A44 B

Triamcinolone is a corticosteroid with significant glucocorticoid effects, which implies that the drug has good anti-inflammatory activity. Compared with hydrocortisone, which is a naturally occurring glucocorticoid secreted by the adrenal cortex, 4 mg of triamcinolone achieve an anti-inflammatory dose equivalent to 20 mg of hydrocortisone. The changes in the chemical structure of triamcinolone that confer an increased anti-inflammatory activity are the formation of cyclic acetonides at the 16 and 17 positions of the glucocorticoid structure and fluorination of the molecule.

Triamcinolone acetonide

A45 B

Ibuprofen is a non-steroidal anti-inflammatory drug which brings about a reduction in the formation of prostaglandins that occur in an inflammatory reaction. Ibuprofen achieves this action by reversibly inhibiting cyclo-oxygenase enzymes. It is a propionic acid derivative.

A46 A

Pseudoephedrine and ephedrine are sympathomimetic agents that stimulate alpha- and beta-adrenergic receptors in the sympathetic nervous system, causing constriction of smooth muscles and blood vessels and producing bronchodilatation. They have central nervous system stimulant activity. Pseudoephedrine is a stereoisomer of ephedrine and it is present as a nasal decongestant in a number of cold and cough preparations, such as Day Nurse.

A47 D

The three products listed are all examples of antipsychotics, with risperidone and quetiapine representing atypical antipsychotics. Long-acting depot injections of antipsychotics are particularly useful where compliance with oral treatment presents a problem and the patient is not stable. Risperidone is available as a depot injection. Quetiapine is available only as tablets, whereas prochlorperazine is available as an injection but is not a long-acting depot preparation.

A48 C

Feldene Melt tablets can be administered by asking the patient to either place the tablet on the tongue, where it will melt, or to swallow the tablet. They dissolve quickly on the tongue, eliminating the disadvantages of dispersible tablets where reconstitution with potable water is necessary. Feldene Melt contains piroxicam, which is an NSAID; as with all NSAIDs, patient should be advised to take the dose with or after food.

A49 C

Isoflurane is a volatile liquid anaesthetic that is administered through calibrated vaporisers using a carrier gas. Isoflurane causes muscle relaxation and it potentiates the effects of muscle relaxant drugs such as atracurium that are also sometimes used in general anaesthesia. Heart rate may rise during isoflurane anaesthesia and there is an increased risk of arrhythmias when it is given with adrenaline.

A50 E

Atenolol is a beta-adrenoceptor blocking drug. Side-effects of atenolol include bradycardia, heart failure and conduction disorders. Cordarone X contains amiodarone, which is an anti-arrhythmic drug. When amiodarone is administered to patients receiving atenolol there is an increased risk of bradycardia, atrioventricular block and myocardial depression. This interaction is considered to be clinically significant and concomitant use should be avoided. Yasmin contains drosperinone (progestogen) and ethinylestradiol (oestrogen). Oestrogens may antagonise hypotensive effect of beta-blockers. When Yasmin and atenolol are used together, blood pressure reduction should be monitored. Deltacortril contains prednisolone, a glucocorticoid. Corticosteroids may antagonise the hypotensive effect of beta-blockers, hence during corticosteroid therapy an elevation in blood pressure at the usual dose of atenolol may be seen. However, the interactions with Yasmin and Deltacortril are not considered to be clinically significant.

A51 B

Plaquenil contains hydroxychloroquine, which is an antimalarial product used in the management of active rheumatoid disease of moderate inflammatory activity. It suppresses the disease process. In long-term treatment, it is associated with visual changes and retinal damage, although to a lesser extent than chloroquine. Before starting treatment, baseline visual acuity should be assessed. During treatment, visual acuity should be monitored annually and the patient should be advised to seek advice if ocular symptoms occur. Methotrexate, which is another disease-modifying anti-rheumatic drug, may present pulmonary fibrosis as a side-effect.

A52   A

All the products should be avoided in severe liver disease. Bezalip contains bezafibrate, which is a fibrate used as a lipid-regulating drug. NovoNorm contains repaglinide, an antidiabetic drug. Septrin contains co-trimoxazole, which consists of trimethoprim and sulfamethoxazole.

A53   A

Co-Diovan consists of valsartan, an angiotensin-II receptor antagonist and hydrochlorothiazide (thiazide diuretic). In diabetic nephropathy, angiotensin-converting enzyme (ACE) inhibitors and angiotensin-II receptor antagonists are used to minimise the risk of renal deterioration and to control blood pressure. Hydrochlorothiazide may be useful in patients with diabetic nephropathy to manage hypertension.

A54   B

Diabetic neuropathy presents with peripheral neuropathy and the patient complains of numbness, muscular pain and weakness. Ibuprofen may be used to relieve mild to moderate pain. Gabapentin, an anti-epileptic drug, is used for the treatment of neuropathic pain, as is amitriptyline and nortriptyline (tricyclic antidepressants). Opioid analgesics may be considered when other drugs have failed. Metoclopramide is used to promote gastric transit in gastroparesis.

A55 A

Levitra contains vardenafil, which is a phosphodiesterase type-5 inhibitor indicated for the management of erectile dysfunction. It causes smooth muscle relaxation. Peak plasma concentrations are achieved within 30–120 minutes and onset of action is expected within 25–60 minutes. It has a low bioavailability of around 15%. Onset of action may be delayed if the drug is administered with a high-fat meal because the rate of absorption is reduced.

A56 B

Syndol is a compound analgesic preparation as it contains paracetamol (non-opioid analgesic) and codeine (opioid analgesic). It also contains caffeine and doxylamine (antihistamine). Doxylamine is a sedating antihistamine. Each tablet of Syndol contains 500 mg paracetamol and the dosage regimen is one to two tablets every 4–6 h.

A57 D

Ikorel contains nicorandil, which is a potassium-channel activator with a nitrate component. It produces arterial and venous vasodilation and is indicated for prophylaxis and treatment of angina. No clinical significant interaction with nifedipine has been reported. When nifedipine and nicorandil are used together, side-effects of vasodilation such as headache and flushing may be more pronounced. Use of nicorandil may bring about a reduction in blood pressure as an unwanted effect and it is contraindicated in hypotension.

A58 E

Metabolism of phenytoin (anti-epileptic drug) is inhibited by clarithromycin (macrolide antibacterial agent) resulting in an increased plasma concentration of phenytoin. Phenytoin accelerates metabolism of doxycycline (tetracycline antibacterial drug) resulting in a reduced plasma concentration of doxycycline.

A59   A

Fosamax contains alendronic acid, a biphosphonate that is associated with oesophageal reactions such as oesophagitis and oesophageal ulcers. For this reason, patients should be advised to swallow tablets whole and with plenty of water while sitting or standing. Xatral XL and Natrilix SR present slow-release preparations, which should be swallowed whole to maintain the slow-release formulation. Xatral XL contains alfuzosin (an alpha-blocker) and Natrilix SR contains indapamide (a diuretic).

A60   C

The use of coal tar in psoriasis is based on its anti-inflammatory properties. However, its pungent smell and messiness compromise its use. It is not harmful to normal skin but irritation and contact allergy may occur.

A61   B

Terbinafine is an allylamine derivative used as an antifungal agent. When used topically, terbinafine clears infection up to four times more quickly than imidazole antifungal agents. Terbinafine is the drug of choice for fungal nail infections.

A62   D

Coversyl contains perindopril, an angiotensin-converting enzyme (ACE) inhibitor. Spironolactone is considered for patients with severe heart failure who are also receiving ACE inhibitors. With spironolactone, close monitoring of serum creatinine and potassium is required. Spironolactone may induce hyperkalaemia. Concomitant use of low-dose spironolactone and perindopril may increase risk of hyperkalaemia, and potassium plasma level should be monitored.

A63 A

When sympathomimetic drugs are used topically for nasal decongestion, they cause a vasoconstricting effect in the nasal mucosa. If used for a prolonged period, rebound congestion occurs, probably because of a compensatory vasodilatation of the tissues. Longer-acting products such as xylometazoline are slower to produce rebound congestion than shorter-acting products such as ephedrine.

A64 C

When suppositories are used for the management of haemorrhoids, there is a probability that they may melt in the rectum, thus bypassing the anal areas. The active ingredients therefore do not reach the inflammation. Creams and ointments are preferred for the management of haemorrhoids.

A65 B

Autoimmune thrombocytopenia purpura is a reduced amount of platelets in the blood. Chronic disease may be presented by scattered petechiae, epistaxis and menorrhagia. Corticosteroids are commonly used to manage the condition. Prednisolone, a corticosteroid with predominantly glucocorticoid activity, is used at a dose of 1 mg/kg daily which is gradually reduced as an increase in the platelet count is achieved.

A66 C

Methylphenidate is an amphetamine-related drug used for the management of attention deficit hyperactivity disorder. Side-effects include insomnia, restlessness, irritability and excitability, nervousness, night terrors and euphoria. Methylphenidate does not generally affect growth as occurs with the amphetamines, but it is still advisable to monitor growth during treatment.

A67   A

Docetaxel is a taxane that is used as an antineoplastic agent. A characteristic side-effect for docetaxel is persistent fluid retention, usually presenting as leg oedema, that may be resistant to treatment. Corticosteroids such as dexamethasone are used to reduce fluid retention.

A68   D

Pegylated liposomal formulations of doxorubicin are available for intravenous use. Doxorubicin is a cytotoxic antibiotic used as an antineoplastic agent and which is associated with dose-related cardiomyopathy. Extravasation during intravenous administration is associated with severe tissue necrosis. The pegylated liposomal formulation of doxorubicin may reduce the incidence of cardiotoxicity and lower the potential for local necrosis.

A69   E

Furosemide is a loop diuretic and sertindole is a selective serotonin re-uptake inhibitor. There is no clinical significant interaction.

A70   D

Mixtard 30 is a mixture of biphasic isophane insulin of human origin and isophane insulin. The proportion is 30% biphasic isophane insulin and 70% isophane insulin.

A71   A

Transient ischaemic attacks (TIAs) are associated with occlusion of the carotid artery and present as brief cerebral disturbances that last less than 24 h and are similar to a stroke. Corrective surgery of the carotid artery to remove occlusion may be beneficial in TIAs. This intervention will limit the development of TIAs into a stroke within a year.

A72 B

Dipyridamole may be used for secondary prevention of transient ischaemic attacks. It may be used in combination with aspirin.

A73 E

After an ischaemic event a single dose of aspirin (antiplatelet drug) 150–300 mg is administered as soon as possible. This dose is followed by a maintenance dose of 75 mg daily. Clopidrogel is another antiplatelet drug that may be used in combination with low-dose aspirin for acute coronary syndrome. Side-effects of clopidrogel include bleeding disorders. Long-term routine concomitant use of aspirin and clopidrogel increases the risk of bleeding.

A74 A

Lithium is used in the prophylaxis and treatment of mania and in the prophylaxis of bipolar disorder and recurrent depression. Perindopril is an angiotensin-converting enzyme (ACE) inhibitor. When perindopril is administered to patients receiving lithium, the ACE inhibitor reduces excretion of lithium resulting in an increased plasma concentration of lithium. Concominant use is not advisable.

A75 D

Zafirlukast is a leukotriene receptor antagonist that is used in the prophylaxis of asthma. The administration of erythromycin (macrolide antibacterial agent) may result in a reduced plasma concentration of zafirlukast. However, this interaction is not considered to be clinically significant and does not warrant avoidance of concomitant administration.

A76   A

Day Nurse contains paracetamol (analgesic and antipyretic), pholcodine (antitussive) and pseudoephedrine (sympathomimetics). Moclobemide is a reversible monoamine-oxidase inhibitor. When Day Nurse is administered to patients receiving moclobemide, the metabolism of pseudoephedrine is inhibited and there is a risk of a hypertensive crisis.

A77   D

Stilnoct contains zolpidem, a non-benzodiazepine hypnotic agent. Dependence has been reported. Side-effects include amnesia, diarrhoea, nausea, vomiting, vertigo, dizziness, headache, drowsiness, asthenia and disturbances of hearing, smell, speech and vision.

A78   C

Lamotrigine and valproate are anti-epileptic agents. In epilepsy, combination therapy may be necessary. Valproate causes an increase in plasma-lamotrigine concentration. This may result in increased side-effects associated with lamotrigine. Side-effects of lamotrigine include rashes, fever, malaise and drowsiness.

A79   C

Effectiveness of combined oral contraceptives may be considerably reduced if drugs that are hepatic enzyme inducers are concurrently used. Both lamotrigine and valproate may be used in tonic-clonic seizures. They are not hepatic enzyme inducers.

A80   E

Breast-feeding is acceptable with some anti-epileptic drugs, such as valproate and carbamazepine, when taken in normal doses as they are present in breast milk in small amounts only.

A81   A

Tavanic contains levofloxacin, which is a quinolone that has activity against Gram-positive and Gram-negative organisms including pneumococci. Quinolones are bactericidal.

A82   E

Guidelines indicate either trimethoprim or amoxicillin or nitrofurantoin or oral cephalosporin as first-line treatment in uncomplicated lower urinary tract infection. Tavanic is available as 250 mg and 500 mg tablets. The cost of a Tavanic 500 mg five-tablet pack is £12.93 and a 10-tablet pack is £25.85.

A83   B

Quinolones are associated with photosensitivity reactions and therefore patient should be advised to avoid excessive exposure to sunlight. Other side-effects of quinolones include nausea, vomiting, dyspepsia, abdominal pain, diarrhoea, headache and dizziness. Patient could be warned that dizziness may occur and that it is preferable to take the drug after meals to reduce nausea.

A84   D

Quinolones may lower the seizure threshold and they should be used with caution in patients with a history of epilepsy or conditions that predispose to seizures. The risk of convulsions is increased if quinolones are administered concomitantly with NSAIDs such as Voltarol (diclofenac). Absorption of levofloxacin may be impaired by antacids. Gaviscon (an antacid) should be taken at a different time from that of levofloxacin. Tofranil contains imipramine, which is a tricyclic antidepressant that does not have a clinically significant drug interaction with levofloxacin.

A85 A

Avelox contains moxifloxacin, a quinolone that is active against Gram-positive and Gram-negative organisms, including pneumococci. Moxifloxacin has a similar spectrum of activity as levofloxacin. Ciproxin contains ciprofloxacin, which is a quinolone that is active against Gram-positive and Gram-negative organisms but it has lower activity against pneumococci compared with levofloxacin. Utinor contains norfloxacin, which is another quinolone. Norfloxacin has lower potency than ciprofloxacin. Fucidin contains fusidic acid, which is a narrow-spectrum antibacterial agent with activity against staphylococci. Klaricid contains clarithromycin, a macrolide antibacterial agent.

A86 E

Daktarin oral gel contains miconazole, an antifungal agent, which, although applied topically, is absorbed to some extent. It is used in the treatment of oral candidiasis and oral fungal infections.

A87 B

Daktarin preparations contain miconazole and are available as cream, powder and spray. Daktarin preparations are not contraindicated in children under 5 years.

A88   B

Patient should be advised to apply the Daktarin oral gel after food and to retain it in the mouth. As with fungal infections, patient should be advised to continue treatment for 2 days after symptoms clear.

A89   D

Dexa-Rhinaspray Duo contains dexamethasone (corticosteroid) and tramazoline, which is a sympathomimetic and acts as an alpha-adrenoceptor agonist.

A90   B

Dexa-Rhinaspray Duo is not recommended for children under 5 years. Side-effects associated with its administration include dryness, irritation of the nose and throat, and nasal bleeding.

A91   C

Zomig contains zolmitriptan, which is a $5HT_1$-agonist used as an anti-migraine drug. It produces vasoconstriction of cranial arteries. Zolmitriptan is metabolised in the liver.

A92   C

The dosage regimen for zolmitriptan is one tablet of 2.5 mg as soon as possible after the onset of an acute migraine attack and this can be repeated after not less than 2 h, if symptoms persist or recur. The maximum dose in 24 h should not exceed 10 mg (four tablets). One of the side-effects associated with the use of zolmitriptan is drowsiness.

A93   B

Zolmitriptan is intended for the treatment of acute migraine attacks. Contraindications to its use include ischaemic heart disease, previous myocardial infarction, coronary vasospasm, previous cerebrovascular accident or transient ischaemic attacks and uncontrolled or severe hypertension.

A94   E

When zolmitriptan is used with St John's wort, increased serotonergic effects may occur and it is advisable to avoid concomitant use. Yasmin, which is a combined hormonal contraceptive, contains drospirenone (progesterone) and ethinylestradiol (oestrogen). Losec, which is a proton pump inhibitor, contains omeprazole. There is no interaction between zolmitriptan and oestrogens, progestogens and proton pump inhibitors.

A95   E

Zomig is presented as tablets in a six-tablet pack that costs £24 and 12-tablet pack that costs £48. Cost per tablet is £4. It is marketed by AstraZeneca.

A96   D

Imigran contains sumatriptan, which is another $5HT_1$-agonist. Migril and Sanomigran are two other anti-migraine drugs that contain an active ingredient that is not a $5HT_1$-agonist. Migril contains ergotamine. Sanomigran contains pizotifen, which is an antihistamine and serotonin antagonist. Syndol and Migraleve are compound analgesics. Syndol contains paracetamol, caffeine, codeine and doxylamine, whereas Migraleve contains paracetamol, codeine and buclizine in the pink tablets.

A97–100

Gaviscon liquid contains sodium alginate, sodium bicarbonate and calcium carbonate. Phillips' Milk of Magnesia contains magnesium hydroxide and Maalox contains magnesium hydroxide and aluminium hydroxide. The symptoms presented by the patient are suggestive of gastro-oesophageal reflux disease, hence an alginate-containing product such as Gaviscon liquid is recommended as first choice. Maalox presents a combination of magnesium and aluminium salts thereby reducing colonic side-effects associated with magnesium and aluminium when used as single agents. Phillips' Milk of Magnesia tends to cause diarrhoea as a side-effect. Sodium bicarbonate is not recommended for use as a single-agent for the relief of dyspepsia.

A97   4

A98   2

A99   1

A100 3

Section 2

Closed-book questions

Test 4

Questions

Questions 1–15

Directions: Each of the questions or incomplete statements is followed by
five suggested answers. Select the best answer in each case.

Q1   Which of the following is the most appropriate for the management of
allergic rhinitis?

A   ☐   pseudoephedrine
B   ☐   promethazine
C   ☐   oxymetazoline
D   ☐   diphenhydramine
E   ☐   levocetirizine

Q2   Advice that could be provided to a patient who wants to increase
appetite includes all of the following EXCEPT:

A   ☐   vary food selections
B   ☐   vary texture of food at meals
C   ☐   garnish meal with herbs
D   ☐   do not consume alcohol
E   ☐   eat frequent small meals

Q3 Which of the following may be recommended for use in a 3-month-old baby with chronic constipation?

A ☐ glycerol suppositories
B ☐ bisacodyl
C ☐ ispaghula husk
D ☐ sodium picosulfate
E ☐ senna

Q4 A drug that is an antagonist is:

A ☐ valsartan
B ☐ lisinopril
C ☐ morphine
D ☐ simvastatin
E ☐ insulin

Q5 Factors that affect drug absorption include all EXCEPT:

A ☐ drug half-life
B ☐ gastric motility
C ☐ blood flow
D ☐ food intake
E ☐ pH at absorption site

Q6 Which of the following is an example of a prodrug?

A ☐ imipramine
B ☐ paracetamol
C ☐ codeine
D ☐ diclofenac
E ☐ paroxetine

Q7   Pharmacoepidemiology:

A   ☐ is the study of the use and effects of drugs in a large number of people

B   ☐ concerns adverse reactions

C   ☐ relates to drug elimination from the body

D   ☐ is the analysis of drug disposition factors

E   ☐ relates to drug wastage

Q8   A patient is prescribed prednisolone 10 mg daily for 16 days. Prednisolone is available as 5 mg enteric coated tablets. How many tablets of Deltacortril have to be dispensed?

A   ☐ 10

B   ☐ 16

C   ☐ 32

D   ☐ 100

E   ☐ 160

Q9   Doxorubicin is available as 25 mL vials at a concentration of 2 mg/mL. The dose required is 200 mg. How many vials are required?

A   ☐ 2

B   ☐ 4

C   ☐ 8

D   ☐ 10

E   ☐ 12

Q10 Betnovate 30 g cream contains 0.1% betamethasone. How many grams of betamethasone are used to prepare the cream:

A ☐ 0.1 g
B ☐ 0.01 g
C ☐ 0.03 g
D ☐ 1 g
E ☐ 3 g

Q11 Timolol 0.25% eye drops is equivalent to how many mg of timolol/mL:

A ☐ 0.0025 mg
B ☐ 0.025 mg
C ☐ 0.25 mg
D ☐ 2.5 mg
E ☐ 25 mg

Q12 Insulin syringes:

A ☐ are calibrated in mL
B ☐ are calibrated in units
C ☐ a large gauge needle is required
D ☐ maximum volume is 5 mL
E ☐ needle length is 10 cm

Q13 Which of the following NSAIDs causes a lower risk of gastrointestinal side-effects?

A ☐ mefenamic acid
B ☐ indometacin
C ☐ piroxicam
D ☐ naproxen
E ☐ celecoxib

Q14   Fluconazole is a (an):

A   ☐   polymyxin antibacterial
B   ☐   protease inhibitor antiviral
C   ☐   triazole antifungal
D   ☐   imidazole antifungal
E   ☐   polyene antifungal

Q15   Isoflurane is a (an):

A   ☐   antimuscarinic
B   ☐   anaesthetic
C   ☐   muscle relaxant
D   ☐   anticholinesterase
E   ☐   benzodiazepine antagonist

Questions 16–35

Directions: Each group of questions below consists of five lettered headings followed by a list of numbered questions. For each numbered question select the one heading that is most closely related to it. Each heading may be used once, more than once or not at all.

Questions 16–20 concern the following drugs:

A   ☐   metronidazole
B   ☐   nitrofurantoin
C   ☐   chloramphenicol
D   ☐   doxycycline
E   ☐   ciprofloxacin

Select, from **A** to **E**, which one of the above:

Q16 requires monitoring of blood count

Q17 has high activity against anaerobic bacteria

Q18 its use as a systemic agent is reserved for life-threatening infections

Q19 is mainly active against Gram-positive and *Escherichia coli*

Q20 intake of alcohol should be avoided during drug therapy

Questions 21–23 concern the following drugs:

A ☐ salbutamol
B ☐ codeine
C ☐ carbocisteine
D ☐ xylometazoline
E ☐ fluticasone

Select, from **A** to **E**, which one of the above is used for:

Q21 nasal congestion

Q22 dry cough

Q23 allergic rhinitis

Questions 24–27 concern the following drugs:

A ☐ diclofenac
B ☐ pseudoephedrine
C ☐ ispaghula husk
D ☐ loperamide
E ☐ codeine

Select, from A to E, which one of the above should be used with caution or is contra-indicated in:

Q24   peptic ulceration

Q25   active ulcerative colitis

Q26   glaucoma

Q27   diabetes

Questions 28–31 concern the following:

A   ☐   thyroglobulin
B   ☐   arachidonic acid
C   ☐   corticotrophin-releasing factor
D   ☐   thromboxane
E   ☐   prostacyclin

Select, from A to E, which one of the above:

Q28   is metabolised by cyclo-oxygenase to produce prostaglandins

Q29   stimulates the release of adrenocorticotrophic hormone

Q30   undergoes iodination in the synthesis of thyroid hormones

Q31   is metabolised by phospholipase A2

Questions 32–35 concern the following drugs:

A   ☐   co-proxamol
B   ☐   co-phenotrope
C   ☐   co-codamol
D   ☐   co-trimoxazole
E   ☐   co-careldopa

Select, from A to E, which one of the above:

Q32 is indicated for parkinsonism

Q33 may be used as an adjunct to rehydration salts in diarrhoea

Q34 is marketed as Septrin

Q35 comprises an extracerebral dopa-decarboxylase inhibitor

Questions 36–60

Directions: For each of the questions below, ONE or MORE of the responses is (are) correct. Decide which of the responses is (are) correct. Then choose

A ☐ if 1, 2 and 3 are correct
B ☐ if 1 and 2 only are correct
C ☐ if 2 and 3 only are correct
D ☐ if 1 only is correct
E ☐ if 3 only is correct

Directions summarised				
A	B	C	D	E
1, 2, 3	1, 2 only	2, 3 only	1 only	3 only

Q36 Diltiazem:

1 ☐ is a calcium-channel blocker
2 ☐ has peripheral and coronary vasodilator properties
3 ☐ has a positive inotropic effect

Q37 Risk factors for hypotension include:

1 ☐ dehydration
2 ☐ sedentary lifestyle
3 ☐ high-fat diet

Q38 Risks of electrolyte imbalance increase in:

1 ☐ older persons
2 ☐ ascites
3 ☐ vomiting

Q39 Enalapril:

1 ☐ is an angiotensin-converting enzyme inhibitor
2 ☐ may have to be withdrawn because of the development of a persistent cough
3 ☐ may cause hypokalaemia

Q40 Drugs that may cause alopecia include:

1 ☐ simvastatin
2 ☐ bleomycin
3 ☐ cisplatin

Q41 Hyperprolactinaemia:

1 ☐ is an excessive prolactin release from the pituitary
2 ☐ may cause infertility
3 ☐ may be drug-induced

Q42   Antibiotic prophylaxis to prevent endocarditis is required before a dental intervention in:

1   ☐ patients with prosthetic cardiac valves
2   ☐ asthmatics
3   ☐ diabetic patients

Q43   Parasympathomimetics:

1   ☐ may cause blurred vision
2   ☐ should be used with caution in asthma
3   ☐ act as miotics

Q44   Nitrazepam:

1   ☐ is less likely to cause a hangover effect than lorazepam
2   ☐ withdrawal syndrome may develop within a few hours of stopping long-term therapy
3   ☐ is used for insomnia

Q45   Myasthenia gravis:

1   ☐ has skeletal muscle weakness as a characteristic symptom
2   ☐ occurs in elderly patients
3   ☐ is treated with atenolol

Q46   Hypromellose:

1   ☐ is used in tear deficiency
2   ☐ has antibacterial properties
3   ☐ should be applied two times daily

Q47 Barrier creams:

1   ☐ protect the skin from becoming macerated
2   ☐ consist of silicones and zinc
3   ☐ may be used to protect against napkin dermatitis

Q48 Hypothyroidism:

1   ☐ onset is insidious in the elderly
2   ☐ requires life-long replacement of thyroxine
3   ☐ radioactive iodine is used

Q49 In diabetic patients:

1   ☐ a random blood glucose level of 20 mmol/L indicates that the
        condition is not being managed properly
2   ☐ low calorie intake is preferred
3   ☐ smoking cessation advice should be provided

Q50 Metformin:

1   ☐ is used in patients who have failed to control blood glucose
        levels on diet
2   ☐ is used in overweight patients because it does not cause
        weight gain
3   ☐ is less likely to cause clinical hypoglycaemia than sulphonyl-
        ureas

Q51 Visceral pain:

1   ☐ may occur in the abdominal viscera
2   ☐ is poorly localised
3   ☐ an example is migraine

Q52 Common causes of nausea and vomiting include:

1 ☐ labyrinthitis
2 ☐ peptic ulcer
3 ☐ infection

Q53 Antiseptics include:

1 ☐ sodium chloride
2 ☐ cetrimide
3 ☐ povidone-iodine

Q54 Constituents of emollient bath additives include:

1 ☐ liquid paraffin
2 ☐ crotamiton
3 ☐ calamine

Q55 Teething gels contain (an):

1 ☐ anaesthetic
2 ☐ antiseptic
3 ☐ acetylsalicyclic acid

Q56 Modified-release oral preparations of iron are:

1 ☐ intended to release iron gradually
2 ☐ administered once daily
3 ☐ associated with a high frequency of gastrointestinal side-effects

Q57 Non-pharmacological measures to control allergic rhinitis include:

1 ☐ washing pets weekly
2 ☐ vacuuming the house regularly
3 ☐ using carpets in all the house

Q58   Positive risk factors for hyperlipidaemia include:

1   ❑ hypertension
2   ❑ diabetes
3   ❑ a high HDL level

Q59   Isosorbide may cause:

1   ❑ dizziness
2   ❑ headaches
3   ❑ postural hypotension

Q60   Magnesium hydroxide:

1   ❑ acts as an antacid as well as a laxative
2   ❑ liquid formulation should be shaken before use
3   ❑ should not be used with a high-fibre diet

Questions 61–80

Directions: The following questions consist of a first statement followed by a second statement in the right-hand column. Decide whether the first statement is true or false. Decide whether the second statement is true or false. Then choose:

A   ❑ if both statements are true and the second statement is a **correct explanation** of the first statement

B   ❑ if both statements are true but the second statement **is NOT a correct explanation** of the first statement

C   ❑ if the first statement is true but the second statement is false

D   ❑ if the first statement is false but the second statement is true

E   ❑ if both statements are false

Directions summarised			
	First statement	**Second statement**	
A	True	True	Second statement is a *correct explanation* of the first
B	True	True	Second statement is *NOT a correct explanation* of the first
C	True	False	
D	False	True	
E	False	False	

Q61 Clarithromycin is a macrolide antibacterial drug. Side-effects include nausea, dyspepsia and loose stools.

Q62 Doses of gabapentin should be taken at evenly spaced times throughout the day. Gabapentin is used to control seizures.

Q63 When applying ear drops for ear wax removal keep the ear tilted for a few minutes after application. Use a cotton bud to remove ear wax.

Q64 Elderly patients are at risk of developing drug-induced oesophagitis. Elderly patients present a delay in oesophageal transit time of medications.

Q65 Amiloride is given in combination with a thiazide diuretic. Amiloride is a weak diuretic that causes potassium retention.

Q66 Steam inhalation is good expectorant therapy. Steam inhalation is not useful for nasal congestion.

Q67 Metoclopramide is a first-line treatment for vomiting during pregnancy. Metoclopramide is not associated with extrapyramidal effects.

Q68 Psoriasis is characterised by epidermal thickening and scaling. Emollients are widely used in psoriasis.

Q69 Imipramine is a tricyclic antidepressant. Imipramine has marked antimuscarinic and cardiac side-effects.

Q70 Buspirone is used as a hypnotic. Buspirone acts at serotonin receptors.

Q71 Low-molecular-weight heparins are only available as subcutaneous injection. Low-molecular-weight heparins have a shorter duration of action than heparin.

Q72 Patients receiving warfarin should not be administered co-trimoxazole. Concominant administration results in an enhanced effect of warfarin.

Q73 Artificial saliva should not contain electrolytes. Artificial saliva should be of neutral pH.

Q74 Corticosteroids should be used with caution in children. Corticosteroids may cause growth retardation.

Q75 Aciclovir can be used for the prophylaxis of cold sores. Cold sores are caused by the herpes virus.

Q76 Calamine lotion is used as first-line treatment of insect bites. Calamine lotion is used against pruritus.

Q77 Fluvastatin should be used with caution in patients with a history of liver disease. Fluvastatin is a fibrate used as a lipid-regulating drug.

Q78 Side-effects associated with atenolol include tachycardia. Atenolol is a sympatholytic agent.

Q79 The difference in anti-inflammatory activity between different NSAIDs is small. Variation in individual patient tolerance and response to NSAIDs exists.

Q80 Anal fissure is a tear in the mucosa of the lower anal canal. It could be associated with haemorrhoids.

Questions 81–85

These questions concern the following structure:

Q81 The structure represents

A ☐ tricyclic antidepressants
B ☐ phenothiazines
C ☐ thioxanthenes
D ☐ butyrophenones
E ☐ dibenzodiazepines

Q82 This class of drugs:

A ☐ acts on the dopamine receptors of the brain
B ☐ may cause dependence
C ☐ may be implicated in food interactions
D ☐ has a narrow therapeutic index
E ☐ may cause Reye's syndrome

Q83 An indication for use is:

A ☐ psychoses
B ☐ epilepsy
C ☐ Parkinson's disease
D ☐ panic disorder
E ☐ obesity

Q84 Adverse reactions to be expected include:

1 ☐ akathisia
2 ☐ drowsiness
3 ☐ dry mouth

A ☐ 1, 2, 3
B ☐ 1, 2 only
C ☐ 2, 3 only
D ☐ 1 only
E ☐ 3 only

Q85 Examples of this class of drugs include:

1 ☐ amitriptyline
2 ☐ chlorpromazine
3 ☐ prochlorperazine

A ☐ 1, 2, 3
B ☐ 1, 2 only
C ☐ 2, 3 only
D ☐ 1 only
E ☐ 3 only

Questions 86–100

Directions: These questions involve prescriptions or patient requests. Read the prescription or patient request and answer the questions.

Questions 86–87: Use the prescription below:

```
┌─────────────────────────────────────────────────────────┐
│                                                           │
│   Patient's name      .................................   │
│                                                           │
│   Proctosedyl ointment                                    │
│   bd    m 1 tube                                          │
│                                                           │
│                                                           │
│                                                           │
│   Doctor's signature   .................................  │
│                                                           │
└─────────────────────────────────────────────────────────┘
```

Q86 Proctosedyl ointment is used:

1 ☐ as an antibacterial
2 ☐ for an anti-inflammatory effect
3 ☐ for an analgesic effect

A ☐ 1, 2, 3
B ☐ 1, 2 only
C ☐ 2, 3 only
D ☐ 1 only
E ☐ 3 only

Q87 The patient should be advised:

1 ☐ to apply ointment morning and evening
2 ☐ to increase fluid intake
3 ☐ to keep applying Proctosedyl regularly

A   ❑ 1, 2, 3
B   ❑ 1, 2 only
C   ❑ 2, 3 only
D   ❑ 1 only
E   ❑ 3 only

Questions 88–92: Use the prescription below:

Patient's name ....
Paroxetine 1 daily   m 28
Doctor's signature ....

Q88   Paroxetine could be used for:

1   ❑ depression
2   ❑ panic disorder
3   ❑ psychoses

A   ❑ 1, 2, 3
B   ❑ 1, 2 only
C   ❑ 2, 3 only
D   ❑ 1 only
E   ❑ 3 only

Q89 Paroxetine is available as:

A ☐ capsules 5 mg
B ☐ capsules 10 mg
C ☐ capsules 20 mg
D ☐ tablets 20 mg
E ☐ tablets 100 mg

Q90 The patient should be advised:

1 ☐ to take medication with food
2 ☐ that medicine may take a few weeks before benefits are experienced
3 ☐ to check their supply before going on holiday

A ☐ 1, 2, 3
B ☐ 1, 2 only
C ☐ 2, 3 only
D ☐ 1 only
E ☐ 3 only

Q91 Common side-effects that could occur include:

1 ☐ abdominal pain
2 ☐ urinary retention
3 ☐ arrhythmias

A ☐ 1, 2, 3
B ☐ 1, 2 only
C ☐ 2, 3 only
D ☐ 1 only
E ☐ 3 only

Q92 Significant interactions could occur if paroxetine is administered concurrently with:

1   ☐ warfarin
2   ☐ promethazine
3   ☐ co-amoxiclav

A   ☐ 1, 2, 3
B   ☐ 1, 2 only
C   ☐ 2, 3 only
D   ☐ 1 only
E   ☐ 3 only

Questions 93–97: Use the prescription below:

Patient's name   ....
Levocabastine nasal spray
2 sprays bd   m 1
Doctor's signature   ....

Q93 Levocabastine is a (an):

A   ☐ corticosteroid
B   ☐ antihistamine
C   ☐ astringent
D   ☐ decongestant
E   ☐ antifungal

Q94 Levocabastine has the following properties:

1 ☐ anti-inflammatory
2 ☐ anti-infective
3 ☐ sympathomimetic

A ☐ 1, 2, 3
B ☐ 1, 2 only
C ☐ 2, 3 only
D ☐ 1 only
E ☐ 3 only

Q95 Levocabastine is used in:

1 ☐ allergic rhinitis
2 ☐ nasal polyps
3 ☐ nasal congestion

A ☐ 1, 2, 3
B ☐ 1, 2 only
C ☐ 2, 3 only
D ☐ 1 only
E ☐ 3 only

Q96 Levocabastine:

1 ☐ is also available as eye drops
2 ☐ is less effective than budesonide
3 ☐ is less effective than cromoglicate

A ☐ 1, 2, 3
B ☐ 1, 2 only
C ☐ 2, 3 only
D ☐ 1 only
E ☐ 3 only

Q97 The patient should be advised:

1 ☐ to apply two puffs into each nostril twice daily
2 ☐ that levocabastine will give symptomatic relief of rhinorrhoea
3 ☐ that sedation occurs commonly

A ☐ 1, 2, 3
B ☐ 1, 2 only
C ☐ 2, 3 only
D ☐ 1 only
E ☐ 3 only

Questions 98–100: For each question read the patient request and answer the question.

Q98 A 40-year-old patient asks for a product to use as a prophylaxis for osteoporosis. Which component should be considered?

A ☐ vitamin C
B ☐ calcium
C ☐ vitamin A
D ☐ folic acid
E ☐ iron

Q99 Constituents of a first-aid spray include:

1 ☐ anaesthetic
2 ☐ antiseptic
3 ☐ corticosteroid

A ☐ 1, 2, 3
B ☐ 1, 2 only
C ☐ 2, 3 only
D ☐ 1 only
E ☐ 3 only

Q100 Contact lens multipurpose solutions:

1 ☐ are specifically available for use with disposable lenses
2 ☐ are sterile solutions
3 ☐ can be used to store lenses

A ☐ 1, 2, 3
B ☐ 1, 2 only
C ☐ 2, 3 only
D ☐ 1 only
E ☐ 3 only

Test 4

Answers

A1   E

Management of allergic rhinitis includes the use of antihistamines, intranasal corticosteroids and nasal decongestants. Non-sedating antihistamines such as levocetirizine are preferred in mild-to-moderate and intermittent symptoms. Promethazine and diphendyramine are sedating antihistamines. Oxymetazoline is a nasal decongestant that is available for topical administration. Topical administration of sympathomimetic agents provides relief from nasal obstruction but because of the onset of rebound congestion their use should be limited to 1 week.

A2   D

Advice on non-pharmacotherapeutic measures to increase appetite includes variation of food at meals, garnishing meals with herbs, variation of food selections and eating frequent small meals. Moderate consumption of alcohol does not impact negatively on appetite.

A3   A

Glycerol suppositories act as a rectal stimulant and may also have some lubricating and softening actions. It is useful in babies and children and acts within 15 to 30 minutes. Bisacodyl, sodium picosulfate and senna are stimulant laxatives that are generally not preferred in children. However, they may be recommended by physicians in children to prevent recurrence of faecal impaction. Ispaghula Husk is a bulk-forming laxative that is not recommended for use in children under 6 years of age.

A4 A

Valsartan is an angiotensin-II receptor antagonist that blocks the actions of angiotensin resulting in lowering of blood pressure. Lisinopril is an angiotensin-converting enzyme (ACE) inhibitor that inhibits the conversion of angiotensin I to angiotensin II. Angiotensin I is an inactive precursor of angiotensin II that has a variety of activities including vasoconstriction. Morphine is an opioid analgesic that acts as an agonist at endorphin receptors. Simvastatin is a statin that acts by competitively inhibiting the enzyme HMG-CoA (3-hydroxy-3-methyl-glutaryl-CoA) reductase that controls the synthesis of cholesterol in the liver. Insulin is a peptide that is normally produced by the pancreas.

A5 A

Drug absorption is affected by gastric motility, blood flow, food intake and pH at absorption site. The half-life of a drug is the time taken for the concentration of the drug to fall to half its original value. It does not affect drug absorption.

A6 C

A prodrug is a substance that needs to be metabolised into a pharmacological active product. Codeine is metabolised in the liver to morphine, norcodeine and other metabolites.

A7 A

Pharmacoepidemiology is the study of use and effects of drugs in large numbers of people. Pharmacovigilance is the monitoring of adverse effects and may be considered to be one aspect of pharmacoepidemiology.

A8   C

Patient requires two tablets of Deltacortril daily. The number that need to be dispensed is two tablets for 16 days = 32 tablets.

A9   B

A vial contains 50 mg of doxorubicin (25 mL × 2 mg). To obtain 200 mg, four vials are required.

A10   C

Betamethasone 0.03 g is required to prepare 30 g of 0.1% betamethasone cream (30 g × 0.1/100).

A11   D

Timolol 2.5 mg/mL is equivalent to a 0.25% timolol eye drop solution. A solution of this strength contains 0.25 g in 100 mL, therefore in 1 mL there is 0.0025 g, which is equal to 2.5 mg.

A12   B

Insulin syringes are calibrated in units. Insulin preparations intended to be administered using the conventional syringe and needle method are presented in units/mL.

A13   E

Celecoxib is a selective of cyclo-oxygenase-2 inhibitor that confers gastro-intestinal tolerance.

A14 C

Fluconazole is a triazole antifungal agent.

A15 B

Isoflurane is a volatile liquid anaesthetic.

A16 C

Chloramphenicol is an antibacterial drug that has a broad spectrum of activity. As it is associated with blood disorders, including reversible and irreversible aplastic anaemia, monitoring of blood counts before and periodically during treatment is required.

A17 A

Metronidazole is an anti-infective agent with high activity against anaerobic bacteria and protozoa.

A18 C

As chloramphenicol is associated with serious haematological side-effects when administered systemically, it is reserved for life-threatening infections.

A19 B

Nitrofurantoin is a bactericidal agent that is active against Gram-positive organisms and *Escherichia coli*. It is indicated in uncomplicated lower urinary tract infections.

A20   A

Intake of alcohol should be avoided during treatment with metronidazole because a disulfiram-like reaction may occur.

A21   D

Xylometazoline is a topical nasal decongestant that is an alpha-adrenoceptor agonist. It causes nasal vasoconstriction and thus relieves congestion.

A22   B

Cough suppressants, also referred to as antitussives, may be recommended in dry cough. Codeine, an opioid drug, suppresses the cough reflex by depressing the cough centres in the brain. Cough suppressants may cause sputum retention.

A23   E

Fluticasone is a corticosteroid that can be used as an intranasal preparation in nasal allergy.

A24   A

Diclofenac is a NSAID and its use is associated with gastrointestinal side-effects including nausea, diarrhoea, bleeding and ulceration. Diclofenac is contraindicated in patients with a history of active peptic ulceration.

A25   D

Ulcerative colitis is a condition characterised by inflammation of the colo-rectal area. Symptoms may include diarrhoea. The use of loperamide in active ulcerative colitis should be undertaken with caution because it may precipitate paralytic ileus and toxic megacolon.

A26 B

Pseudoephedrine is a sympathomimetic agent and should be avoided in patients with conditions of raised intraocular pressure such as glaucoma.

A27 B

Pseudoephedrine is a sympathomimetic agent and it is not suitable for patients with diabetes because of its metabolic effects on blood glucose and because of its vasoconstrictor effects, which may lead to hypertension. Diabetic patients are already prone to hypertension.

A28 B

Arachidonic acid is metabolised by the cyclo-oxygenase group of enzymes to produce prostaglandins.

A29 C

Corticotrophin-releasing factor is released by the hypothalamus to stimulate the pituitary gland to release adrenocorticotrophic hormone.

A30 A

Thyroglobulin is a protein that undergoes iodination in the thyroid gland leading to the synthesis of thyroid hormones.

A31   B

Phospholipase A2 is an enzyme that mediates a deacylation reaction of arachidonic acid.

A32   E

Co-careldopa is a mixture of levodopa and carbidopa (dopa-decarboxylase inhibitor). Levodopa is used in parkinsonism to replenish the depleted striatal dopamine.

A33   B

Co-phenotrope is a mixture of diphenoxylate and atropine. Diphenoxylate is an antimotility drug that can be used in diarrhoea.

A34   D

Co-trimoxazole consists of a mixture of two anti-bacterial agents, trimethoprim and sulfamethoxazole. An example of a proprietary name for this mixture is Septrin, marketed by GlaxoSmithKline.

A35   E

Co-careldopa includes carbidopa, which is an extracerebral dopa-decarboxylase inhibitor. It reduces the peripheral conversion of levodopa to dopamine, resulting in a greater amount of levodopa reaching the brain. Effective brain-dopamine concentrations are achieved with lower doses of levodopa than if levodopa were used as a single agent.

A36 B

Diltiazem is a calcium-channel blocker, specifically a benzothiazipine derivative. All calcium-channel blockers have peripheral and coronary vasodilator
properties. Diltiazem has a negative inotropic effect as a cardiac effect,
although less than verapamil.

A37 D

Hypotension occurs when the blood pressure is below a 'normal' value (usually
a diastolic below 70–80 mmHg). Dehydration may lead to hypotension. A
sedentary lifestyle and high-fat diet are contributory factors for hypertension.

A38 A

Risks for electrolyte imbalance include being elderly, presence of ascites and
vomiting. There are a number of factors that predispose older patients to a
higher risk of electrolyte imbalance. These include drug therapy such as
diuretics, ACE inhibitors, NSAIDs and antacids. Older persons may be taking
a number of different drugs that impact on electrolyte balance. Elderly patients
may also have a reduced fluid intake. Ascites is the accumulation of fluid in
the peritoneal cavity resulting in a disruption of the osmotic and water balance.
Vomiting leads to electrolyte and water loss.

A39 B

Enalapril is an angiotensin-converting enzyme (ACE) inhibitor. ACE inhibitors
are associated with a persistent cough as a side-effect. Sometimes this side-
effect impacts negatively on the patient's lifestyle and warrants withdrawal of
treatment. ACE inhibitors, through their inhibition of angiotensin II formation,
result in a reduction of aldosterone release. As a result, ACE inhibitors have
potassium-sparing effects. Treatment with enalapril may result in hyperkalaemia.

A40   A

Alopecia is loss of hair and this condition may occur as a consequence to drug therapy. Simvastatin is a statin that may also cause alopecia, along with other side-effects associated with statins. Cytotoxic drugs such as bleomycin (cytotoxic antibiotic) and cisplatin (platinum compound) may cause varying degrees of hair loss.

A41   A

Hyperprolactinaemia is an excessive prolactin release from the pituitary gland. It is characterised by infertility in patients. Drugs that may cause hyperprolactinaemia include phenothiazines, haloperidol, methyldopa, cimetidine, metoclopramide and oestrogens. Prolactin produces mammary gland enlargement and induces milk production.

A42   D

Antibiotic prophylaxis is recommended in patients who are at special risk of endocarditis, namely patients with prosthetic cardiac valves or patients who have had endocarditis previously.

A43   A

Parasympathomimetics such as pilocarpine are used in eye preparations for the management of glaucoma because of their miotic activity. Ocular side-effects include blurred vision. As parasympathomimetics result in bronchoconstriction, they should be used with caution in patients with asthma.

A44   E

Nitrazepam is a benzodiazepine that is used as a hypnotic in the short-term management of insomnia. Nitrazepam has a long half-life and therefore it is associated with more hangover effects than shorter acting products such as lorazepam. Withdrawal phenomena are more common with shorter acting products because the residual concentration of nitrazepam delays the onset of withdrawal symptoms.

A45   D

Myasthenia gravis is characterised by skeletal muscle weakness. It is a neuromuscular disorder that can occur at any age. Treatment includes use of anticholinesterases, corticosteroids and immunosuppressants such as azathioprine.

A46   D

Hypromellose is a mixed cellulose ether that is used for tear deficiency. It lubricates the eye and prevents dryness caused by tear deficiency. It is applied as required to achieve adequate relief.

A47   A

Barrier preparations provide a mechanical block which protects the skin from irritants, thus preventing maceration. They consist of silicones and zinc salts. Regular application of barrier preparations to the napkin area prevents napkin dermatitis.

A48   B

Hypothyroidism is a condition associated with the failure of the thyroid gland to produce enough thyroid hormone. Incidence of hypothyroidism increases with age and symptoms in the elderly are quite insidious. Life-long replacement of thyroxine is required to maintain thyroid hormone levels. Radioactive iodine is a treatment option in the management of hyperthyroidism.

A49 A

Random glucose levels should be maintained at less than 11.1 mmol/L. Higher levels indicate that the patient is not being managed properly. HbA1c testing is appropriate in detecting long-term control of blood glucose. Diabetic patients are advised to follow a low-calorie diet and to adopt a healthier lifestyle by, for example, stopping smoking and taking more exercise.

A50 A

Metformin is a bigaunide antidiabetic agent that is used when strict dieting has failed to control diabetes or when other treatment options have failed. It is preferred in overweight patients because it does not cause weight gain, which may occur with sulphonylureas. Hypoglycaemia does not usually occur with metformin because, unlike sulphonylureas, it does not stimulate or mimic insulin.

A51 B

Visceral pain occurs in the internal organs, commonly in the abdominal organs. It is usually poorly localised. Migraine is a neurovascular condition associated with disturbances in the cranial-blood circulation.

A52 A

Nausea and vomiting are symptoms of conditions that include vestibular disorders such as labyrinthitis, gastrointestinal conditions such as peptic ulceration and infection.

A53 A

Examples of antiseptics include sodium chloride (saline), cetrimide and povidone-iodine.

A54 D

Emollient bath additives are intended to hydrate the skin and are used for dry skin conditions. Constituents include liquid paraffin, which is a greasy preparation. Crotamiton and calamine are antipruritics.

A55 B

Teething gels contain an anaesthetic such as lidocaine and an antiseptic such as cetalkonium, found in Bonjela gel. Acetylsalicylic acid is aspirin and is not recommended for use in children.

A56 B

Modified-release oral preparations release the active ingredient gradually over time. This also applies to modified-release oral preparations of iron. They are intended for once-daily dosage. Compared with the normal oral dosage formulations, the modified-release preparations of iron are associated with a lower incidence of gastrointestinal irritation (nausea, epigastric pain). This may reflect the smaller amount of iron that is successfully absorbed with a modified-release preparation.

A57 B

Symptoms of allergic rhinitis may be reduced by controlling dust and animal dander in the house. This may be achieved by washing pets weekly, by using a vacuum cleaner regularly and by not using carpets in the home.

A58 B

Conditions that may contribute or exacerbate hyperlipidaemia include hypertension and diabetes. A raised low-density lipoprotein (LDL) cholesterol level is associated with atherogenesis and a raised high density lipoprotein (HDL) cholesterol level is associated with a low risk of hyperlipidaemia. LDL carries cholesterol from the gastrointestinal tract, liver or tissues for storage whereas HDL transports cholesterol from the tissues to the liver for breakdown.

A59   A

Isosorbide is a nitrate used in the management of angina and left ventricular failure. It is a potent vasodilator and side-effects associated with its use include dizziness, throbbing headache, flushing and postural hypotension.

A60   B

Magnesium hydroxide reacts with gastric acid thus neutralising it. It is useful as an antacid. It tends to be laxative and in higher doses it can be used as an osmotic laxative. Magnesium hydroxide, when presented as a liquid formulation, tends to precipitate and the consumer is advised to shake it before use.

A61   B

Clarithromycin is an erythromycin derivative. Gastrointestinal side-effects include nausea, vomiting, dyspepsia and diarrhoea.

A62   B

Gabapentin is an anti-epileptic drug that is usually prescribed as three divided doses. Taking the drug at evenly spaced times throughout the day achieves a better drug plasma profile, avoiding high peak-plasma concentrations that may contribute to adverse effects, or low plasma concentrations that may lead to seizures.

A63 C

When applying ear drops, the patient should be advised to keep the ear tilted for a few minutes after application to avoid drug loss through seepage. The use of cotton buds should be discouraged in ear wax removal because they may damage the tympanic membrane.

A64 A

Older patients are at risk of developing drug-induced oesophagitis because drugs and other factors may result in delayed oesophageal transit time of medications.

A65 A

Amiloride is a weak diuretic but its characteristic is that it causes potassium retention. When used in combination with thiazide diuretics, amiloride counteracts the potassium loss attributed to thiazide diuretics.

A66 C

Steam inhalation is useful in the management of the symptoms of acute respiratory tract infection. It encourages the inspiration of warm, moist air in the bronchi, which is comforting in nasal congestion as an expectorant therapy.

A67 E

Metoclopramide is an anti-emetic agent that is usually recommended for the management of vomiting during pregnancy as a second-line treatment after an antihistamine drug such as promethazine has been used unsuccessfully. Metoclopramide resembles phenothiazines in activity and it is also associated with extrapyramidal effects, especially in children and in young adults.

A68 B

Psoriasis is an inflammatory skin condition that is characterised by epidermal thickening and scaling. Emollients are used widely in psoriasis to hydrate the skin and remove the itchiness.

A69 B

Imipramine is a tricyclic antidepressant drug that is associated with antimuscarinic and cardiac side-effects. Antimuscarinic side-effects include dry mouth, sedation, blurred vision and constipation. Cardiac side-effects include electrocardiographic changes, arrhythmias, postural hypotension and tachycardia.

A70 D

Buspirone is used short-term as an anxiolytic. It acts at serotonin receptors.

A71 C

Low-molecular-weight heparins (LMWHs) are administered by subcutaneous injection. They are as effective as unfractionated heparin in the prevention of venous thrombo-embolism. An advantage of LMWHs is that they are administered once daily because they have a longer duration of action than unfractionated heparin.

A72 A

Co-trimoxazole consists of sulfamethoxazole (a sulphonamide) and trimethoprim. Co-trimoxazole should not be administered to patients receiving warfarin because sulphonamides enhance the effect of warfarin.

A73   D

Artificial saliva should be of a neutral pH and consists of electrolytes including fluoride.

A74   A

Corticosteroids should be used with caution in children because pharmaco-therapeutic doses of corticosteroids may retard or interrupt their growth.

A75   D

Aciclovir is an anti-viral drug intended to be used in the management of cold sores. It is recommended for use with the onset of early symptoms, preferably prodromal ones. However, it is not indicated as a prophylactic agent against recurrent cold sores. Cold sores are caused by the virus herpes simplex.

A76   D

The administration of topical hydrocortisone and antihistamines is recommended as first-line treatment in insect bites because they are intended to counteract the inflammatory process. Calamine lotion may be used as an adjunct product for its soothing and antipruritic activity.

A77   C

Fluvastatin is a lipid-regulating drug that is classified as a statin. Statins are contraindicated in patients with active liver disease and should be used with caution in patients with a history of liver disease. Liver function tests should be carried out before initiation of treatment and should be monitored regularly during treatment.

A78 D

Atenolol is a beta-adrenoceptor blocking agent that acts as an antagonist at the sympathetic nervous system. It is a sympatholytic agent and is used as an antihypertensive. Side-effects include bradycardia, caused by its sympatholytic activity.

A79 B

Differences in anti-inflammatory activity between different NSAIDs are small. Variation lies in the individual patient's tolerance and response to the various drugs.

A80 B

Anal fissure is a tear in the epithelial lining of the anal canal. The condition may be precipitated by hard stools and constipation. Patients may present with haemorrhoids and anal fissure as a result of chronic constipation.

A81 B

The structure represents phenothiazines. It is a three-ring structure consisting of two benzene rings that are linked by a sulphur and a nitrogen atom.

A82 A

Phenothiazines have dopamine antagonist properties as well as anticholinergic and H_1-blocking effects.

A83 A

Phenothiazines are used as antipsychotic agents. Some phenothiazines are also used in the management of nausea and vomiting.

A84 A

Side-effects of phenothiazines include extrapyramidal symptoms that consist of parkinsonian symptoms, dystonia, akathisia and tardive dyskinesia and side-effects, such as drowsiness and dry mouth, related to their antimuscarinic activity.

A85 C

Chlorpromazine and prochlorperazine are two examples of phenothiazines. Chlorpromazine has an aliphatic side chain on the R_1 position whereas prochlorperazine has a piperazine group. This results in differences in potency and in the side-effect profile. Amitriptyline is a tricyclic antidepressant.

A86 C

Proctosedyl ointment consists of cinchocaine, which is a local anaesthetic and hydrocortisone, a corticosteroid. It has anti-inflammatory and analgesic properties.

A87 B

The patient has been prescribed Proctosedyl, to be applied twice daily. The patient can be advised to apply the ointment morning and evening and to increase fluid intake so as to avoid hard stools and straining at stools. As Proctosedyl contains a corticosteroid component, it should be used only during the acute phase and for short-term use.

A88 B

Paroxetine is a selective serotonin re-uptake inhibitor, which is used for depression, obsessive-compulsive disorder, panic disorders, social phobia, post-traumatic stress disorder and generalised anxiety disorder. SSRIs should not be used during a manic phase.

A89   D

Available solid oral dosage forms of paroxetine are tablets at 20 mg and 30 mg strengths.

A90   A

Side-effects of paroxetine include gastrointestinal disorders such as nausea, vomiting and dyspepsia. To reduce onset of these side-effects, patient should be advised to take the drug with food. Effectiveness of drug therapy with paroxetine may be delayed until 4–6 weeks. Patient should be advised to check their supply of medication, especially before going on holiday because this is a prescription-only product and treatment should not be withdrawn abruptly.

A91   D

Common side-effects associated with paroxetine administration do not usually include side-effects caused by antimuscarinic activity or cardiovascular disorders. Common side-effects are related to the gastrointestinal tract and include abdominal pain.

A92   D

The anticoagulant effect of warfarin is possibly increased by SSRIs. Paroxetine is not reported to have significant interactions with promethazine and co-amoxiclav.

A93 B

Levocabastine is an antihistamine preparation.

A94 D

As an antihistamine, levocabastine has anti-inflammatory properties.

A95 D

Levocabastine is used in the management of allergic rhinitis.

A96 B

Levocabastine is also available as eye drops for use in allergic conjunctivitis. Topical levocabastine is less effective than topical corticosteroids such as budesonide but more effective than cromoglicate.

A97 B

The patient should be advised to apply two sprays into each nostril twice daily. Levocabastine will relieve the symptoms of allergic rhinitis. Sedation is rare, because it is administered topically.

A98 B

Calcium supplementation is used in the prevention of osteoporosis.

A99   B

First-aid spray preparations include an anaesthetic to counteract the presentation of pain and an antiseptic agent to prevent infection of the injury site.

A100 C

Different contact lens multipurpose solutions are available for soft and hard contact lenses. Soft contact lenses are also available as disposable lenses for short-term use (around 4 weeks) or for once-only wear. Multipurpose solutions are recommended for disposable soft lenses. The multipurpose solution is a sterile preparation that may be used to store lenses.

Test 5

Questions

Questions 1–15

Directions: Each of the questions or incomplete statements is followed by five suggested answers. Select the best answer in each case.

Q1   Causes of cough include all of the following EXCEPT:

A   ☐ anxiety
B   ☐ congestive heart failure
C   ☐ hypertension
D   ☐ chronic bronchitis
E   ☐ enalapril

Q2   Patients should be advised not to consume any alcohol if taking:

A   ☐ co-amoxiclav
B   ☐ amitriptyline
C   ☐ atenolol
D   ☐ bendroflumethiazide
E   ☐ naproxen

Q3   A drug for which abrupt withdrawal is associated with adverse reactions caused by receptor up-regulation is:

A   ☐ pseudoephedrine
B   ☐ prednisolone
C   ☐ pantoprazole
D   ☐ piroxicam
E   ☐ propranolol

Q4 A drug that acts as a 5-hydroxytryptamine receptor antagonist is:

A ☐ cinnarizine

B ☐ promethazine

C ☐ hyoscine

D ☐ ondansetron

E ☐ betahistine

Q5 The volume of distribution of a drug describes:

A ☐ the apparent distribution of the drug in the body

B ☐ the concentration of the drug in plasma

C ☐ the volume of plasma that is cleared from the body

D ☐ the concentration of the drug in blood

E ☐ the rate of elimination of the drug from the body

Q6 A patient is prescribed gentamicin 130 mg every 8 h. Gentamicin is available as 40 mg/mL. The volume needed for one dose is:

A ☐ 0.4 mL

B ☐ 1 mL

C ☐ 3.25 mL

D ☐ 10 mL

E ☐ 32 mL

Q7 Convert 18 μg to milligrams:

A ☐ 18 000

B ☐ 1800

C ☐ 0.0018

D ☐ 0.018

E ☐ 0.18

Q8   A solution of sodium chloride contains 500 mg of sodium chloride made up to 100 mL with water. Express this solution as a percentage w/v:

A   ❑ 500
B   ❑ 50
C   ❑ 5
D   ❑ 0.5
E   ❑ 0.05

Q9   When 500 mL of a 10% ammonia solution are diluted to 1000 mL, the percentage v/v is:

A   ❑ 20
B   ❑ 10
C   ❑ 5
D   ❑ 0.5
E   ❑ 0.05

Q10   The paediatric dose for clarithromycin is 7.5 mg/kg body weight. What is the appropriate dose for a child weighing 25 kg:

A   ❑ 0.19 g
B   ❑ 7.5 mg
C   ❑ 1.9 g
D   ❑ 0.019 g
E   ❑ 0.01 g

Q11 The number of tablets of amitriptyline 25 mg required to prepare 60 mL of a paediatric preparation containing amitriptyline 10 mg per millilitre is:

A ☐ 150
B ☐ 60
C ☐ 10
D ☐ 24
E ☐ 4

Q12 300 mL cisplatin are being administered over 5 h. How many mL/min are given:

A ☐ 0.01
B ☐ 1
C ☐ 5
D ☐ 25
E ☐ 60

Q13 Ointments:

A ☐ are soluble in water
B ☐ contain a high proportion of zinc
C ☐ are not occlusive
D ☐ are suitable for chronic, dry lesions
E ☐ are protective against UVB

Q14 An example of a skeletal muscle relaxant is:

A ☐ baclofen
B ☐ naloxone
C ☐ probenecid
D ☐ orphenadrine
E ☐ trihexyphenidyl

Q15 The cautionary label 'Do not take milk, indigestion remedies or medicines containing iron or zinc at the same time of day as this medicine' is applicable to all the drugs EXCEPT:

A ☐ oxytetracycline
B ☐ tetracycline
C ☐ demeclocycline
D ☐ norfloxacin
E ☐ clarithromycin

Questions 16–35

Directions: Each group of questions below consists of five lettered headings followed by a list of numbered questions. For each numbered question select the one heading that is most closely related to it. Each heading may be used once, more than once or not at all.

Questions 16–19 concern the following parameters:

A ☐ ALP
B ☐ ALT
C ☐ LDL
D ☐ HDL
E ☐ ATP

Select, from A to E, which one of the above:

Q16 is an indicator of cholestasis

Q17 high levels indicate hyperlipidaemia

Q18 is highly elevated in acute hepatitis

Q19 removes cholesterol from local sites

Questions 20–23 concern the following drugs:

A   ☐   alendronate
B   ☐   zolmitriptan
C   ☐   codeine
D   ☐   omeprazole
E   ☐   co-trimoxazole

Select, from A to E, which one of the above should be used with caution or is contra-indicated in the following conditions:

Q20   blood disorders

Q21   decreased respiratory reserve

Q22   ischaemic heart disease

Q23   active gastrointestinal bleeding

Questions 24–28 concern the following:

A   ☐   Factor VIII
B   ☐   angiotensin II
C   ☐   bradykinin
D   ☐   cyclic adenosine monophosphate
E   ☐   substance P

Select, from A to E, which one of the above:

Q24   inhibits release of inflammatory mediators resulting in bronchodilatation

Q25   stimulates aldosterone release

Q26   is produced by injured tissues as a mediator of inflammation

Q27   is a vasoconstrictor

Q28   is a neuropeptide involved in pain transmission and in the release of pro-inflammatory agents

Questions 29–31 concern the following drugs:

A   ☐ xylometazoline
B   ☐ cetirizine
C   ☐ promethazine
D   ☐ desloratidine
E   ☐ levocetirizine

Select, from A to E, which one of the above:

Q29   is available for topical application

Q30   may be used in insomnia

Q31   may be used in motion sickness

Questions 32–35 concern the following drugs:

A   ☐ latanoprost
B   ☐ betaxolol
C   ☐ dipivefrine
D   ☐ dorzolamide
E   ☐ pilocarpine

Select, from A to E, which one of the above:

Q32   is a pro-drug of adrenaline

Q33   is a prostaglandin analogue

Q34   is a mydriatic

Q35   results in a small pupil

Questions 36–60

Directions: For each of the questions below, ONE or MORE of the responses is (are) correct. Decide which of the responses is (are) correct. Then choose:

A   ☐ if 1, 2 and 3 are correct
B   ☐ if 1 and 2 only are correct
C   ☐ if 2 and 3 only are correct
D   ☐ if 1 only is correct
E   ☐ if 3 only is correct

Directions summarised				
A	**B**	**C**	**D**	**E**
1, 2, 3	1, 2 only	2, 3 only	1 only	3 only

Q36   Symptoms of diabetes include:

1   ☐ polyuria
2   ☐ polydipsia
3   ☐ unexplained weight loss

Q37   Obesity:

1   ☐ is common in people with type 2 diabetes
2   ☐ causes insulin resistance
3   ☐ is classified according to the body mass index

Q38   Albuminuria:

1   ☐ is the presence in urine of abnormally large quantities of albumin
2   ☐ is also referred to as proteinuria
3   ☐ may be a sign of diabetic nephropathy

Q39   Drugs that impair glucose tolerance include:

1   ☐ estradiol
2   ☐ codeine
3   ☐ paroxetine

Q40   Sorbitol:

1   ☐ is a monosaccharide
2   ☐ is found in diabetic foods
3   ☐ does not offer benefit over sucrose in weight-reduction diets

Q41   Omega-3 fatty acids:

1   ☐ should be avoided by patients with hyperlipidaemia
2   ☐ are found in fish oils
3   ☐ are available as capsules

Q42   Elderly patients who are administered chlorpromazine are at an increased risk of:

1   ☐   urinary retention
2   ☐   tardive dyskinesia
3   ☐   constipation

Q43   Dysphagia may occur in patients who have:

1   ☐   stroke
2   ☐   Parkinson's disease
3   ☐   Alzheimer's disease

Q44   Clinical presentation of lung cancer includes:

1   ☐   nasal congestion
2   ☐   wheeze
3   ☐   haemoptysis

Q45   Paroxetine:

1   ☐   may be associated with withdrawal symptoms
2   ☐   is used in mania
3   ☐   is contraindicated if the patient has had a recent myocardial infarction

Q46   Antibacterial agent(s) that may be prescribed in salmonellosis include:

1   ☐   erythromycin
2   ☐   cefaclor
3   ☐   ciprofloxacin

Q47 Prophylaxis for meningococcal meningitis includes use of:

1　☐　gentamicin
2　☐　nitrofurantoin
3　☐　rifampicin

Q48 Dexamethasone:

1　☐　lacks mineralocorticoid activity
2　☐　may be used in cerebral oedema
3　☐　is marketed as Deltacortril

Q49 Wax removal ear drops may contain:

1　☐　arachis oil
2　☐　paradichlorobenzene
3　☐　benzyl benzoate

Q50 Anti-inflammatory preparations that are available for ocular administration include:

1　☐　antazoline
2　☐　betamethasone
3　☐　emedastine

Q51 Calcium dietary requirements are relatively greater in:

1　☐　pregnancy
2　☐　childhood
3　☐　diarrhoea

Q52 Clarithromycin should not be administered with:

1　☐　simvastatin
2　☐　spironolactone
3　☐　atenolol

Q53 Prochlorperazine:

1 ☐ is used in vertigo
2 ☐ is a phenothiazine associated with pronounced extrapyramidal symptoms
3 ☐ may cause drowsiness

Q54 Drugs that should be avoided or used with caution in an elderly patient with chronic heart failure include:

1 ☐ clomipramine
2 ☐ thyroxine
3 ☐ perindopril

Q55 Indapamide:

1 ☐ should be avoided in diabetic patients
2 ☐ causes a reduction in circulating fluid volume
3 ☐ is available as a modified-release preparation

Q56 Drugs used in the control of epilepsy include:

1 ☐ valproate
2 ☐ gabapentin
3 ☐ haloperidol

Q57 Extravasation:

1 ☐ causes severe local tissue necrosis
2 ☐ hydrocortisone may be administered to treat the inflammation
3 ☐ may be caused by influenza vaccine

Q58   Cytotoxic antibiotics include:

1   ☐   bleomycin
2   ☐   doxorubicin
3   ☐   mitoxantrone

Q59   Levocetirizine:

1   ☐   is an active metabolite of cetirizine
2   ☐   cannot be taken in combination with sympathomimetics
3   ☐   one tablet daily is the dosage regimen for adults

Q60   Antibacterial agents that can be given to adults at a dosing schedule of an oral formulation twice daily include:

1   ☐   co-amoxiclav
2   ☐   ceftazidime
3   ☐   flucloxacillin

Questions 61–80

Directions: The following questions consist of a statement in the left-hand column followed by a second statement in the right-hand column. Decide whether the first statement is true or false. Decide whether the second statement is true or false. Then choose:

A   ☐   if both statements are true and the second statement is a **correct explanation** of the first statement

B   ☐   if both statements are true but the second statement **is NOT a correct explanation** of the first statement

C   ☐   if the first statement is true but the second statement is false

D   ☐   if the first statement is false but the second statement is true

E   ☐   if both statements are false

Directions summarised			
	First statement	**Second statement**	
A	True	True	Second statement is a *correct explanation* of the first
B	True	True	Second statement is *NOT a correct explanation* of the first
C	True	False	
D	False	True	
E	False	False	

Q61 Topical steroids are very effective and safe in the treatment of eczema. Potent steroids such as hydrocortisone butyrate are used to bring the condition under control.

Q62 Terbinafine is a fungicidal. Terbinafine is used at a stat dose in vaginal candidiasis.

Q63 Antihistamines are used topically for the management of nasal allergies. Antihistamines remove the symptoms of rhinorrhoea, sneezing and nasal obstruction.

Q64 Haloperidol is used as an antipsychotic agent in the management of aggressive patients. Haloperidol has a low incidence of hypotension.

Q65 Amitriptyline increases neuronal uptake of noradrenaline. When amitriptyline is compared with imipramine, it is preferred in patients who are anxious and agitated.

Q66 Clozapine is associated with reduced extrapyramidal effects compared with chlorpromazine. Clozapine is used as a drug of first choice in schizophrenia.

Q67 Iron-deficiency anaemia is characterised by insomnia and hyperactivity. Iron-deficiency anaemia occurs due to G6PD deficiency.

Q68   Antacids will cause immediate relief from a gastric ulcer. Antacids can be used one hour after food.

Q69   Repaglinide is administered at meal times. Repaglinide has a rapid onset of action and a short duration of activity.

Q70   The 'economy-class syndrome' describes DVT leading to pulmonary embolism associated with prolonged travel. It is associated with excess alcohol consumption and dehydration.

Q71   Amlodipine leads to vasoconstriction. A side-effect that may occur with amlodipine is ankle oedema.

Q72   Loperamide is an opioid that does not penetrate the blood–brain barrier. Loperamide should not be recommended for children under 4 years.

Q73   Hyperbilirubinaemia gives rise to jaundice and associated pruritus. Jaundice is the accumulation of fluid in the peritoneal cavity.

Q74   Sore throats may indicate drug-induced neutropenia. Drug-induced neutropenia may be caused by co-trimoxazole.

Q75   The use of a spacer with beclometasone metered dose inhaler may increase steroid-induced oral candidiasis. The spacer should be washed out and left to dry.

Q76   Breath-actuated inhalers are less suitable for children. With breath-actuated inhalers there is no need to coordinate actuation with inhalation.

Q77   An HRT preparation with oestrogen alone is suitable for continuous use in women without a uterus. HRT increases the risk of venous thrombo-embolism and stroke.

Q78   In the elderly, orphenadrine is the mainstay of therapy for the treatment of Parkinson's disease. Orphenadrine is preferred because of a lower incidence of confusion.

Q79 Osteoporosis is a condition that is not presented in males. Osteoporosis may occur because of decreased oestrogen levels.

Q80 Domperidone acts at the chemoreceptor trigger zone and does not readily cross the blood-brain barrier. Domperidone can be given three times daily.

Questions 81–85

These questions concern the following structure:

Q81 The structure represents a drug that is a (an):

A ☐ beta-blocker
B ☐ anticholinergic
C ☐ cholinergic agonist
D ☐ serotonin antagonist
E ☐ antihistamine

Q82 An indication for use is:

A ☐ angina
B ☐ nausea and vomiting
C ☐ Parkinson's disease
D ☐ allergy
E ☐ depression

Q83   The drug:

A   ☐   acts primarily on the gastrointestinal tract
B   ☐   should be used with caution in diabetic patients
C   ☐   competitively antagonises bradykinin
D   ☐   initial dose should be given at bedtime
E   ☐   should not be administered with bendroflumethiazide

Q84   Side-effects to be expected include:

1   ☐   bronchospasm
2   ☐   dry mouth
3   ☐   weight loss

A   ☐   1, 2, 3
B   ☐   1, 2 only
C   ☐   2, 3 only
D   ☐   1 only
E   ☐   3 only

Q85   Contraindications to its use include:

1   ☐   angina
2   ☐   glaucoma
3   ☐   asthma

A   ☐   1, 2, 3
B   ☐   1, 2 only
C   ☐   2, 3 only
D   ☐   1 only
E   ☐   3 only

Questions 86–100

Directions: These questions involve prescriptions or patient requests. Read the prescription or patient request and answer the questions.

Questions 86–88: Use the prescription below:

Patient's name ....

Fucithalmic 1% viscous eye drops
2 drops bd

Doctor's signature ....

Q86 A characteristic of Fucithalmic preparation is that:

A ❑ it has a broad spectrum of activity
B ❑ it is a sustained-release formulation
C ❑ it presents a systemic method of drug administration
D ❑ it contains a steroid component
E ❑ it is presented as single-application packs

Q87 How many milligrams of active ingredient are present per gram of Fucithalmic:

A ❑ 0.01
B ❑ 1
C ❑ 10
D ❑ 100
E ❑ 1000

Q88   The patient should be advised:

1   ☐   to apply two drops morning and evening
2   ☐   that transient stinging may occur
3   ☐   to place applicator on lower lid margin and squeeze container

A   ☐   1, 2, 3
B   ☐   1, 2 only
C   ☐   2, 3 only
D   ☐   1 only
E   ☐   3 only

Questions 89–90: Use the prescription below:

Patient's name   ....

Micralax micro-enema
prn   m 4

Doctor's signature   ....

Q89   Micralax is a laxative that is classified as:

A   ☐   osmotic
B   ☐   stimulant
C   ☐   bulk-forming
D   ☐   bowel cleanser
E   ☐   antispasmodic

Q90 Micralax:

1   ❑ may be used in a 4-year-old child
2   ❑ may be used when there is infrequent defecation
3   ❑ each unit contains one litre

A   ❑ 1, 2, 3
B   ❑ 1, 2 only
C   ❑ 2, 3 only
D   ❑ 1 only
E   ❑ 3 only

Questions 91–93: Use the prescription below:

Patient's name   ....
Bumetanide 5 mg
daily   m 30
Doctor's signature   ....

Q91 Bumetanide:

1   ❑ is similar in activity to furosemide
2   ❑ is indicated for oedema
3   ❑ is a mild diuretic

A   ❑ 1, 2, 3
B   ❑ 1, 2 only
C   ❑ 2, 3 only
D   ❑ 1 only
E   ❑ 3 only

Q92   The patient is advised:

1   ☐ to take three tablets daily
2   ☐ to take the medication at night
3   ☐ that the medication will act within one hour

A   ☐ 1, 2, 3
B   ☐ 1, 2 only
C   ☐ 2, 3 only
D   ☐ 1 only
E   ☐ 3 only

Q93   Which supplement should be considered in patients taking bumetanide?

A   ☐ sodium
B   ☐ potassium
C   ☐ glucose
D   ☐ zinc
E   ☐ calcium

Questions 94–97: Use the prescription below:

Patient's name   ....
Flagyl tablets
200 mg tds
Augmentin 625 mg tablets
bd
Doctor's signature   ....

Q94 The above prescription is most likely to be prescribed when the patient presents with symptoms of:

1. ☐ dental infection
2. ☐ systemic mycoses
3. ☐ tinea pedis infection

A. ☐ 1, 2, 3
B. ☐ 1, 2 only
C. ☐ 2, 3 only
D. ☐ 1 only
E. ☐ 3 only

Q95 The patient is advised:

1. ☐ to take Augmentin tablets twice daily
2. ☐ to take Flagyl tablets with or after food
3. ☐ to take tablets at regular intervals

A. ☐ 1, 2, 3
B. ☐ 1, 2 only
C. ☐ 2, 3 only
D. ☐ 1 only
E. ☐ 3 only

Q96 Flagyl:

1. ☐ is only available as 400 mg tablets
2. ☐ may cause an unpleasant taste as a side-effect
3. ☐ contains metronidazole

A. ☐ 1, 2, 3
B. ☐ 1, 2 only
C. ☐ 2, 3 only
D. ☐ 1 only
E. ☐ 3 only

Q97 Augmentin:

1   ☐ includes amoxicillin
2   ☐ absorption is not affected by the presence of food in the stomach
3   ☐ should not be used in infections likely to be caused by beta-lactamase producing strains

A   ☐ 1, 2, 3
B   ☐ 1, 2 only
C   ☐ 2, 3 only
D   ☐ 1 only
E   ☐ 3 only

Questions 98–100: For each question read the patient request.

Q98 A 45-year-old patient with a history of peptic ulcer disease asks for an analgesic for a headache. Which product could be recommended?

A   ☐ ibuprofen
B   ☐ co-codamol
C   ☐ aspirin
D   ☐ naproxen
E   ☐ meloxicam

Q99 A patient requests aspirin 75 mg tablets. Aspirin 75 mg:

1   ☐ decreases platelet aggregation
2   ☐ is available as enteric coated tablets
3   ☐ should be avoided in patients with a history of a coronary bypass surgery

A ☐ 1, 2, 3
B ☐ 1, 2 only
C ☐ 2, 3 only
D ☐ 1 only
E ☐ 3 only

Q100 A patient requests a topical antipruritic agent. The preparation may consist of:

A ☐ desloratidine
B ☐ white soft paraffin
C ☐ dimeticone
D ☐ calcipotriol
E ☐ crotamiton

Test 5

Answers

A1   C

Hypertension is not associated with onset of cough. Congestive heart failure is associated with shortness of breath, oedema and cough. Chronic bronchitis presents with wheezing and cough. Symptoms of anxiety may be varied and include dyspnoea, palpitations, cough. Enalapril is an angiotensin-converting enzyme inhibitor that may be associated with cough.

A2   B

Amitriptyline is a tricyclic antidepressant that, when administered with alcohol, may result in an increased sedative effect.

A3   E

Propranolol is a beta-adrenoceptor blocking agent. The antagonist effect is associated with up-regulation of receptors. Once the drug is withdrawn abruptly, adverse reactions may occur due to the up-regulation of the receptors.

A4   D

Ondansetron is an antagonist at the 5-hydroxytryptamine receptor ($5HT_3$ antagonist) within the serotonergic system. Cinnarizine, promethazine and betahistine are antihistamines. Hyoscine is an antimuscarinic agent.

A5   A

Volume of distribution is an important parameter in clinical pharmacokinetics. It describes the apparent distribution of the drug in the body. It refers to the fluid volume required to contain the drug in the body at the same concentration as in blood or plasma.

A6   C

Forty milligrams are available in 1 mL; 130 mg are therefore available in 3.25 mL (130/40).

A7   D

Eighteen micrograms are equivalent to 0.018 milligrams.

A8   D

The solution contains 0.5 g in 100 mL, % w/v is 0.5.

A9   C

In 100 mL of the 10% ammonia solution, 10 g of ammonia are available. Hence in 500 mL, 50 g are present (500 × 10/100). Therefore when 500 mL of solution are diluted to 1000 mL, 50 g are present in 1000 mL. The %v/v is 5 (100 × 50/1000).

A10   A

The appropriate dose for a child weighing 25 kg is 187.5 mg (7.5 × 25), which is equivalent to 0.19 g.

A11   D

In 60 mL of a 10 mg/mL amitriptyline solution, 600 mg of amitriptyline are present. Therefore 24 tablets are required to make up this solution (600/25).

A12   B

Three hundred millilitres are administered over 300 minutes resulting in a 1 mL/min administration rate.

A13   D

Ointments are greasy preparations that are usually insoluble in water and are more occlusive than creams. These characteristics make them suitable for chronic, dry lesions.

A14   A

Baclofen is a skeletal muscle relaxant. Naloxone is an antagonist for central and respiratory depression. Probenecid is a uricosuric drug. Orphenadrine and trihexyphenidyl are antimuscarinic agents used in parkinsonism.

A15   E

Clarithromycin is a macrolide drug. Absorption of clarithromycin is not affected by milk, iron or zinc. Norfloxacin is a quinolone and the other products are tetracyclines. Absorption of norfloxacin and tetracyclines may be affected if taken at the same time as milk or medicines containing iron or zinc.

A16   A

Cholestasis is interference with the flow of bile. This results in build-up in the liver of products that are usually excreted in bile. These products include alkaline phosphatase (ALP).

A17 C

Raised levels of low-density lipoprotein (LDL) cholesterol are associated with hyperlipidaemia.

A18 B

Hepatitis is an inflammatory condition of the liver characterised by hepato-cellular necrosis. In the acute phase, this results in large elevations in alanine transaminase (ALT) and aspartate transaminase (AST). Elevations in alkaline phosphatase (ALP) are slight.

A19 D

High-density lipoprotein (HDL) is a carrier that takes up cholesterol from local sites.

A20 E

Co-trimoxazole is a mixture of antibacterial agents that contains trimethoprim and sulfamethoxazole. Co-trimoxazole is associated with rare but serious side-effects, including blood disorders such as neutropenia, thrombocytopenia, agranulocytosis and purpura. For this reason, co-trimoxazole should be used with caution or is avoided in patients with blood disorders.

A21 C

Codeine is an opioid drug that in large doses may cause respiratory depression. For this reason, it should be used with caution in patients with decreased respiratory reserve.

A22   B

Zolmitriptan is a $5HT_1$-agonist that is used as an antimigraine drug. $5HT_1$-agonists may cause coronary vasoconstriction, which may present as chest tightness and, on rare occasions, it may result in severe cardiovascular events. For this reason, this class of drugs is contraindicated in ischaemic heart disease.

A23   A

Alendronate is a biphosphonate drug that is used in the management of osteoporosis. It may precipitate oesophageal reactions such as oesophagitis, oesophageal ulcers and oesophageal erosions. For this reason, it is used with caution or may be contraindicated in active gastrointestinal bleeding.

A24   D

Cyclic adenosine monophosphate (cyclic AMP) in the bronchial airways results in inhibition of release of inflammatory mediators such as histamine and this in turn results in bronchodilatation.

A25   B

Angiotensin II is converted from angiotensin I by angiotensin-converting enzymes. Angiotensin I is formed from angiotensinogen, a protein produced by the liver. Angiotensin II stimulates aldosterone release from the adrenal gland.

A26   C

Bradykinin is produced through a proteolytic reaction by injured tissues as a mediator of inflammation. Bradykinin produces vasodilation resulting in increased capillary permeability and oedema. It is broken down by angiotensin-converting enzymes.

A27   B

Angiotensin II is a vasoconstrictor that causes a rise in blood pressure.

A28   E

Substance P is a polypeptide that acts as a neurotransmitter in pain transmission and initiates processes that result in the release of pro-inflammatory agents such as leukotrienes and prostaglandins.

A29   A

Xylometazoline is a sympathomimetic agent that is available as a topical application in the form of nasal drops or a spray for nasal congestion and in eye drops for allergic conjunctivitis.

A30   C

Promethazine is a sedating antihistamine that may be used in the management of insomnia.

A31   C

Promethazine is an antihistamine that may be used as a prophylactic agent in motion sickness.

A32 C

Dipivefrine is a pro-drug of adrenaline that presents more rapid penetration through the cornea than adrenaline (epinephrine). It is used as a sympatho-mimetic agent in the treatment of glaucoma. It reduces production of aqueous humour and increases outflow through the trabecular mesh.

A33 A

Latanoprost is a prostaglandin analogue that is available as a topical agent for the treatment of glaucoma. It increases outflow and results in a reduction in intraocular pressure.

A34 C

Sympathomimetics dilate the pupil, a mydriatic action. Consequently dipive-frine may precipitate angle-closure glaucoma in susceptible persons. For this reason, dipivefrine is contraindicated in patients with angle-closure glaucoma.

A35 E

Pilocarpine is a miotic agent and hence causes a small pupil effect. It is used in the management of glaucoma but the miotic effect is an unwanted side-effect that may cause discomfort because of reduced visual acuity, reduced night vision and frontal headache.

A36 A

Diabetes is a metabolic disorder that may have an insidious onset, especially for type 2 diabetes. Symptoms related to hyperglycaemia include polyuria (excessive urine production) and polydipsia (excessive thirst). Unexplained weight loss caused by impaired glucose utilisation is another presenting symptom of diabetes, especially type 1 diabetes.

A37   A

Obesity is common in type 2 diabetes, which usually presents in later life, whereas type 1 diabetes is associated with early age at onset and with weight loss. Obesity has a bearing on the management of the condition. In patients with type 2 diabetes who can be managed by oral antidiabetics, metformin is used because it does not cause weight gain. In patients requiring insulin, obesity may cause insulin resistance requiring higher doses. Obesity is classified according to the body mass index (BMI).

A38   A

Albumin is a protein that is usually present in trace amounts in the urine. Albuminuria is the presence in the urine of abnormally large quantities of albumin and is a type of proteinuria. It is a prognostic marker for the development of renal disorders associated with filtration problems, which may occur as a consequence of diabetes (diabetic nephropathy) and hypertension.

A39   D

Estradiol is an oestrogen and it may cause glucose intolerance.

A40   A

Sorbitol is a monosaccharide that is used as a sweetener in energy-reduced diabetic foods. It has half the sweetening power of sucrose. It is poorly absorbed from the gastrointestinal tract. However, once absorbed it is metabolised to fructose and glucose. It does not offer benefits over sucrose in weight reduction diets because the amounts used to achieve the equivalent sweetening effect are greater and it still carries calorific content. The intake of sorbitol may be associated with diarrhoea.

A41   C

Omega-3 fatty acids are useful in the treatment of severe hypertriglycerid-aemia and may be used as an adjunct to diet or to drug therapy. They are found in fish oils and are available as capsules or liquid for oral administration.

A42   A

Chlorpromazine is an aliphatic phenothiazine that is associated with pronounced sedative and moderate antimuscarinic effects (such as urinary retention and constipation) and extrapyramidal effects (such as tardive dyskinesia). Older patients may be more prone to develop these side-effects because of prostatic hyperplasia (in males), erratic diet, reduced mobility and parkinsonism, and other drugs that precipitate extrapyramidal effects. Older patients are also more susceptible to hypotension.

A43   A

Dysphagia is a condition where the patient presents with difficulty in swallowing. It may be associated with disorders of the nervous system, such as Parkinson's disease and cerebrovascular accidents (stroke). Alzheimer's disease is a condition associated with progressive dementia.

A44   C

The clinical presentation of lung cancer varies but cough is usually a primary symptom. The tumour may lead to excess sputum production in the bronchial tree leading to wheezing. Haemoptysis (blood-stained sputum) may also occur.

A45   D

Paroxetine is a selective serotonin re-uptake inhibitor (SSRI) used in depressive illness and anxiety disorders. Abrupt withdrawal should be avoided because it is associated with symptoms that include headache, nausea, paraesthesia, dizziness and anxiety. Paroxetine should not be used in a manic phase because it may precipitate the disorder, and should be used with caution in patients with a history of mania. SSRIs are less cardiotoxic than other antidepressants, such as the tricyclic antidepressants (TCAs). They should be used with caution in patients with a history of myocardial infarction but they are preferred to TCAs.

A46   E

Salmonellosis is a gastrointestinal tract infection caused by *Salmonella* species. The quinolone ciprofloxacin or trimethoprim are the recommended antibacterial agents used in the management of salmonellosis.

A47   E

Meningococcal meningitis is a medical emergency. It is a condition caused by the organism *Neisseria meningitidis*. To prevent the spread of infection, people who are in close contact with patients presenting with meningococcal meningitis are prescribed antibacterial agents for prophylactic management. The antibacterial agents recommended for prophylaxis of meningococcal meningitis include rifampicin, ciprofloxacin and ceftriaxone.

A48   B

Dexamethasone is a corticosteroid with high glucocorticoid activity but with insignificant mineralocorticoid activity. It is associated with less fluid retention when used at high doses, compared with products with mineralocorticoid activity. It may be used in the management of cerebral oedema associated with malignancy. Deltacortril contains prednisolone, another corticosteroid.

A49 B

Wax removal preparations contain oil-based products, such as arachis oil, or organic products, such as paradichlorobenzene. Benzyl benzoate is an irritant that is used in the treatment of scabies.

A50 A

Topical anti-inflammatory preparations for ocular use include antazoline and emedastine (antihistamines) and betamethasone (corticosteroid).

A51 B

During pregnancy and in childhood, calcium requirements are relatively greater than during adult years. Calcium dietary intake is important. During diarrhoea, salts and water are lost. However, calcium dietary requirements do not vary.

A52 D

Clarithromycin is a macrolide antibacterial agent. It should not be administered concomitantly with simvastatin (lipid-regulating drug, statin) because it increases risk of myopathy associated with simvastatin.

A53 A

Prochlorperazine is a piperazine phenothiazine that is used in nausea and vomiting, vertigo, labyrinthine disorders, schizophrenia and other psychoses.

It is associated with extrapyramidal symptoms and the frequency of these side-effects is greater with piperazine phenothiazines than with aliphatic and piperazine phenothiazines. Drowsiness may occur with phenothiazines, including prochlorperazine.

A54   B

Clomipramine is a tricyclic antidepressant that should be used with caution in patients with cardiac disease because it is associated with cardiovascular side-effects, such as arrhythmias, tachycardia and syncope. Antidepressant therapy in older patients is associated with hyponatraemia symptoms, including drowsiness, confusion and convulsions. Thyroxine is used as a thyroid hormone in hypothyroidism. It should be used with caution in older persons and in patients with cardiac disease because treatment may precipitate cardiovascular events including anginal pain, arrhythmias and tachycardia. Perindopril is an angiotensin-converting enzyme inhibitor that may be used in the management of heart failure.

A55   C

Indapamide is a thiazide-related diuretic used in the management of hypertension. A characteristic of indapamide is that it causes less aggravation of diabetes mellitus than thiazide diuretics. Indapamide is not contraindicated in diabetic patients. As a diuretic, indapamide results in inhibition of sodium and water re-absorption resulting in a reduction in circulating fluid volume. Indapamide is presented as tablets and modified-release tablets.

A56   B

Valproate and gabapentin are anti-epileptic agents. Valproate is recommended as a first-line drug in different presentations of epilepsy whereas gabapentin is usually reserved for second-line treatment. Haloperidol is a butyrophenone antipsychotic agent with anti-emetic activities. It is used in schizophrenia and related psychoses, anxiety disorders, nausea and vomiting, particularly associated with drug therapy in palliative care. As with other antipsychotics, it may lower the convulsion threshold; haloperidol should be used with caution or avoided in patients with epilepsy.

A57   B

Extravasation occurs when drugs, with either an acidic or alkaline pH or with an osmolarity greater than plasma, leak from the veins during intravenous administration into the subcutaneous or subdermal tissues. It causes severe local tissue necrosis. Hydrocortisone may be administered at the site of extravasation or intravenously to counteract the inflammation occurring with extravasation. Influenza vaccine is administered as a subcutaneous or intramuscular injection and is not associated with extravasation.

A58   A

Bleomycin, doxorubicin and mitoxantrone are cytotoxic antibiotics.

A59   E

Levocetirizine is an isomer of cetirizine. It is an antihistamine that may be recommended together with topical or systemic administration of sympathomimetic agents in the management of nasal allergy. The dosage regimen for adults and children over 6 years is one 5 mg tablet daily.

A60   D

Co-amoxiclav is a mixture of amoxicillin and clavulanic acid. It is available as Augmentin 625 mg tablets that can be given to adults at a dosing schedule of twice daily. Ceftazidime is a cephalosporin that is only available for parenteral administration. Flucloxacillin is a penicillinase-resistant penicillin that is administered to adults at a dosing schedule of every 6 h.

A61 B

Topical corticosteroids are used in the management of eczema because they reduce the inflammatory response. Hydrocortisone, which is a mild steroid, is usually the first-line agent. Hydrocortisone butyrate is a potent steroid that may be used short-term in acute flare-ups to bring the condition under control.

A62 C

Terbinafine is an allylamine derivative used as an antifungal agent. It has fungicidal activity against dermatophytes. It is used in the treatment of dermatophyte infections of the skin and nails and in ringworm infections. It is not indicated for topical or systemic use in the management of vaginal candidiasis.

A63 C

Antihistamines administered topically may be used in the management of nasal allergies. They remove the symptoms of rhinorrhoea, itching and sneezing but not nasal obstruction.

A64 B

Haloperidol is an antipsychotic agent that is useful in the management of schizophrenia, psychomotor agitation, excitement and violent or dangerously impulsive behaviour. It is associated with a high incidence of extrapyramidal effects and tends to cause less hypotension than chlorpromazine.

A65 D

Amitriptyline is a tricyclic antidepressant that inhibits neuronal re-uptake of noradrenaline in the central nervous system. Imipramine is a less sedating antidepressant than amitriptyline. Consequently amitriptyline may be preferred in patients who are anxious and agitated.

A66 C

Clozapine is an atypical antipsychotic characteristically associated with fewer extrapyramidal symptoms than the other antipsychotics. However, clozapine can cause agranulocytosis and for this reason its use is restricted when other treatment options have failed.

A67 E

Iron-deficiency anaemia is due to inadequate iron supply or to iron loss. Characteristic symptoms of anaemia are fatigue, general weakness, drowsiness and pallor. Glucose-6-phosphate dehydrogenase (G6PD) deficiency may cause haemolytic anaemia, which is characterised by increased destruction of red blood cells.

A68 B

Antacid preparations provide effective and immediate relief from a gastric ulcer. Liquid formulations have a faster onset of action. However, antacids do not provide any healing of the condition. They are most effective when taken 1 h after food.

A69 A

Repaglinide is a meglitinide analogue used as an antidiabetic agent. It stimulates insulin release. It should be administered at meal times because it has a rapid onset and a short duration of activity. It is intended to stimulate post-prandial insulin secretion so as to decrease peaking of blood-glucose after meals, and thus avoid hyperglycaemia.

A70   B

The 'economy-class syndrome' is a condition whereby deep-vein thrombosis (DVT) leading to pulmonary embolism is associated with prolonged travel. The risk increases with immobility, excess alcohol consumption and dehydration.

A71   D

Amlodipine is a dihydropyridine calcium-channel blocker with a long duration of action. Calcium-channel blockers cause peripheral and coronary vasodilation. This activity may lead to unwanted effects associated with peripheral vasodilation, such as ankle oedema and flushing.

A72   B

Loperamide is an opioid drug used as an antimotility agent for the management of diarrhoea. It does not penetrate the blood–brain barrier and hence it is very unlikely to be associated with central opioid effects such as respiratory depression. However, loperamide is not recommended for use in children under 4 years. Rehydration therapy should be the mainstay of therapy in children.

A73   C

Hyperbilirubinaemia is the condition of increased levels of bilirubin in plasma. It gives rise to jaundice, which characteristically presents with pruritus. Jaundice is the yellow discoloration of skin, sclera and mucous membranes.

A74   B

Neutropenia is a decreased number of neutrophils. Symptoms of acute neutropenia are fever, sore throat and painful mucosal ulcers. Neutropenia may be drug-induced. Co-trimoxazole, which consists of trimethoprim and sulfamethoxazole, may precipitate blood disorders, including neutropenia.

A75   D

The administration of corticosteroids by inhalation is associated with oral candidiasis. The use of a spacer decreases the deposit of beclometasone on the oral mucosa and therefore lowers risk of oral candidiasis. Proper hygiene of the spacer is required. It should be cleaned once a month by washing with a mild detergent, rinsed and left to dry in air.

A76   B

In children a metered-dose inhaler with a spacer is preferred to breath-actuated inhalers. Improper respiratory function may lead to difficulties in using breath-actuated inhalers. The advantage of breath-actuated inhalers is that there is no need to coordinate actuation with inhalation as is necessary with metered-dose inhalers. The disadvantage of metered-dose inhalers is overcome through the use of a spacer.

A77   B

A hormone replacement therapy (HRT) that contains oestrogen component alone is suitable for continuous therapy in women without a uterus. In women with a uterus, a progestogen component for at least the last 12–14 days of the cycle, to reduce the risk of endometrial cancer, is recommended. HRT preparations are associated with a greater risk of venous thromboembolism and stroke.

A78   E

Orphenadrine is an antimuscarinic agent that may be used in parkinsonism. It is useful in drug-induced parkinsonism but in idiopathic disease it has a moderate effect in reducing symptoms of tremor associated with the condition. Levodopa is considered the mainstay of treatment in elderly patients with Parkinson's disease. Side-effects of orphenadrine include dry mouth, gastro-intestinal disturbances, dizziness, blurred vision as well as confusion, excitement and agitation.

A79   D

Osteoporosis is a metabolic bone disease that occurs in males and females; however, it is more common in women. It is related to oestrogen levels: decreased levels, such as during the menopause, are associated with an increased risk of osteoporosis.

A80   B

Domperidone is a drug used in nausea and vomiting. It acts at the chemo-receptor trigger zone; its advantage is that it does not readily cross the blood–brain barrier. It is less likely to cause the central effects, such as sedation and dystonic reactions, that may be expected with other drugs used in the management of nausea and vomiting, such as metoclopramide and prochlorperazine. Domperidone may be administered three to four times daily.

A81   A

The chemical structure corresponds to atenolol, a beta-adrenoceptor blocking agent.

A82   A

Atenolol is used in hypertension, angina and arrhythmias.

A83 B

Atenolol acts by blocking the beta-adrenoceptor receptors in the cardiovascular system. Beta-adrenoceptor blockers interfere with the sympathetic nervous system that is involved with carbohydrate metabolism. Beta-adrenoceptor blockers interfere with carbohydrate metabolism and insulin regulation. For this reason, they should be used with caution in diabetes because they may precipitate hypoglycaemia and hyperglycaemia. When atenolol is administered with bendroflumethiazide, an increased hypotensive effect may occur. However, co-administration need not be avoided.

A84 D

Side-effects to be expected include bradycardia, heart failure, hypotension, bronchospasm and peripheral vasoconstriction.

A85 E

Contraindications to the use of atenolol include asthma, uncontrolled heart failure, marked bradycardia, hypotension and severe peripheral arterial disease.

A86 B

Fucithalmic contains fusidic acid, which is a narrow-spectrum antibacterial agent active mainly against staphylococcal infections. It is presented as viscous eye drops that provide a sustained-release effect.

A87 C

Fucithalmic contains 1 g fusidic acid in 100 g. Therefore 1 g contains 10 mg (1000 mg/100 g).

A88 B

The patient has been prescribed two drops twice daily. As expected with administration of eye drops, transient stinging may occur. The patient should be advised not to touch the applicator with the lower lid margin.

A89 A

Micralax contains sodium citrate, sodium alkylsulphoacetate, sorbic acid in glycerol and sorbitol. It is an osmotic laxative.

A90 B

Micralax is a micro-enema where each unit presents 5 mL. It may be used in adults and children over 3 years and is indicated in constipation.

A91 B

Bumetanide is a loop diuretic with similar activity to furosemide. It is rapid in action. Diuresis is dose related and may be drastic. It is indicated for oedema.

A92 E

The patient has been prescribed one 5 mg tablet daily, which should be taken during the day. It acts within 1 h and if taken at night the resulting diuresis may disturb sleep.

A93 B

Bumetanide inhibits reabsorption of salts and water from the loop of Henle. Hypokalaemia may develop and therefore potassium supplementation is required to avoid this condition, which may have serious sequelae.

A94 D

Flagyl contains metronidazole, which is effective against anaerobic bacteria and protozoa whereas Augmentin contains co-amoxiclav, a penicillin. This combination is particularly useful in dental infections where there is a probability of mixed infections with anaerobic species.

A95 A

The patient has been prescribed Augmentin tablets twice daily and should be advised to take Flagyl tablets three times daily with or after food and to take the tablets at regular intervals.

A96 C

Flagyl tablets (metronidazole) are available as 200 mg and 400 mg strengths. A characteristic side-effect of metronidazole is that it may cause an unpleasant taste.

A97 B

Augmentin consists of amoxicillin and clavulanic acid, with the latter acting as a beta-lactamase inhibitor. Absorption of amoxicillin is not affected by the presence of food in the stomach.

A98 B

Co-codamol consists of paracetamol and codeine and may be recommended to this patient. All the other products suggested are non-steroidal anti-inflammatory drugs and these are contraindicated in patients with a history of peptic ulcer disease.

A99   B

Low-dose aspirin has an antiplatelet effect because it decreases platelet aggregation. Aspirin 75 mg is available as enteric coated tablets and is given as a prophylactic agent in cerebrovascular disease or myocardial infarction in patients who are at risk, such as those with a history of coronary bypass surgery.

A100   E

Crotamiton is an antipruritic agent that is available for topical administration. Desloratidine is an antihistamine available for systemic use. White soft paraffin is used as a base in a number of preparations. Dimeticone is used as an anti-flatulent agent or may be included in topical barrier preparations. Calcipotriol is a vitamin D analogue and is used in psoriasis.

Test 6

Questions

Questions 1–15

Directions: Each of the questions or incomplete statements is followed by five suggested answers. Select the best answer in each case.

Q1   Within the pharmaceutical industry, the department which ensures that the facilities and systems adopted are adequate is:

A   ☐ research and development department
B   ☐ analytical methods department
C   ☐ production department
D   ☐ quality assurance department
E   ☐ quality control department

Q2   The following vitamins are fat soluble EXCEPT:

A   ☐ vitamin A
B   ☐ vitamin C
C   ☐ vitamin D
D   ☐ vitamin E
E   ☐ vitamin K

Q3   Excessive alcohol consumption may result in all of the following EXCEPT:

A   ☐ memory impairment
B   ☐ vasodilation
C   ☐ dehydration
D   ☐ sensitivity to light
E   ☐ dry mouth

Q4 Cathecol-O-methyltransferase:

A ☐ is only available in the brain
B ☐ causes diffusion of catecholamines into the synaptic cleft
C ☐ causes methylation of norepinephrine
D ☐ causes deamination of norepinephrine
E ☐ causes hydrolysis of norepinephrine

Q5 Which of the following compounds is included with levodopa so that a lower dose can be used to achieve an effective brain-dopamine concentration?

A ☐ pergolide
B ☐ carbidopa
C ☐ selegiline
D ☐ entacapone
E ☐ amantadine

Q6 How many millilitres of a 1 in 500 v/v solution are required to produce 2 L of a 1 in 1000 v/v solution?

A ☐ 100
B ☐ 200
C ☐ 500
D ☐ 1000
E ☐ 2000

Q7 How many grams of salicylic acid are required to prepare 30 g of 2% salicylic acid in aqueous cream?

A ☐ 0.2
B ☐ 0.6
C ☐ 1
D ☐ 2
E ☐ 6

Q8   Calculate the amount of calamine required to prepare 60 g of a cream containing 10% calamine, 15% zinc oxide, aqueous cream to 100 g:

A   ❑ 4
B   ❑ 5
C   ❑ 6
D   ❑ 7
E   ❑ 8

Q9   How many millilitres of 100 units/mL soluble insulin should be administered to achieve a dose of 20 units?

A   ❑ 0.002
B   ❑ 0.02
C   ❑ 0.2
D   ❑ 2
E   ❑ 20

Q10   Pivmecillinam is prescribed at 20 mg/kg in three divided doses. The individual dose (mg) to be administered to a patient weighing 12 kg is:

A   ❑ 8
B   ❑ 80
C   ❑ 240
D   ❑ 800
E   ❑ 2400

Q11 Filgrastim is available as 300 μg per mL injection. A patient with a body weight of 95 kg is prescribed 5 μg/kg daily. How many millilitres are required to present the daily dose?

A ☐ 0.1
B ☐ 1
C ☐ 1.58
D ☐ 15.8
E ☐ 158

Q12 If disodium pamidronate 60 mg is diluted to 250 mL in sodium chloride solution, the millilitres required per minute to deliver 60 mg at a rate of not more than 1 mg/minute over 90 minutes are:

A ☐ 1
B ☐ 2
C ☐ 4
D ☐ 6
E ☐ 10

Q13 A patient requires a dose of 800 μg of dopamine. Dopamine is available as an injection containing 40 mg/mL. The volume in millilitres of the injection required is:

A ☐ 0.002
B ☐ 0.02
C ☐ 0.2
D ☐ 2
E ☐ 20

Q14 With 30 g of sodium chloride, the number of litres of 0.9% saline solution that can be prepared are:

A ☐ 0.03
B ☐ 0.3
C ☐ 3.33
D ☐ 33
E ☐ 330

Q15 When 1 mg of potassium permanganate is dissolved in 500 mL water, the percentage w/v is:

A ☐ 0.001
B ☐ 0.0002
C ☐ 0.002
D ☐ 0.2
E ☐ 2

Questions 16–35

Directions: Each group of questions below consists of five lettered headings followed by a list of numbered questions. For each numbered question select the one heading that is most closely related to it. Each heading may be used once, more than once or not at all.

Questions 16–19 concern the following drugs:

A ☐ pergolide
B ☐ prochlorperazine
C ☐ venlafaxine
D ☐ diazepam
E ☐ lorazepam

Select, from A to E, which one of the above:

Q16 is a dopamine antagonist

Q17 is a short-acting benzodiazepine

Q18 is a noradrenaline re-uptake inhibitor

Q19 is a dopamine receptor agonist

Questions 20–23 concern the following drugs:

A ☐ orlistat
B ☐ omeprazole
C ☐ domperidone
D ☐ senna
E ☐ sibutramine

Select, from A to E, which one of the above can cause:

Q20 oily leakage from rectum

Q21 extrapyramidal effects

Q22 tachycardia

Q23 hypertension

Questions 24–28 concern the following:

A ☐ bendroflumethiazide
B ☐ amiloride
C ☐ indapamide
D ☐ spironolactone
E ☐ furosemide

Select, from A to E, which one of the above:

Q24   is an anthranilic acid derivative with a sulfonamide moiety

Q25   acts prinicipally at the ascending limb of the loop of Henle

Q26   is a competitive inhibitor of aldosterone

Q27   may cause gynaecomastia

Q28   has a fast onset of action

Questions 29–31 concern the following compounds:

A   ☐ ascorbic acid
B   ☐ salicylic acid
C   ☐ aluminium chloride hexahydrate
D   ☐ zinc oxide
E   ☐ heparinoid

Select, from A to E, which one of the above has the following action:

Q29   astringent

Q30   keratolytic

Q31   antiperspirant

Questions 32–35 concern the following drugs:

A   ☐ fluconazole
B   ☐ ketoconazole
C   ☐ itraconazole
D   ☐ miconazole
F   ☐ nystatin

Select, from A to E, which one of the above:

Q32 is indicated as first-line systemic treatment for onchomycosis in the toenails

Q33 is available as a shampoo

Q34 is not available in solid, oral dosage forms

Q35 should be administered with caution to patients at high risk of heart failure

Questions 36–60

Directions: For each of the questions below, ONE or MORE of the responses is (are) correct. Decide which of the responses is (are) correct. Then choose:

A ☐ if 1, 2 and 3 are correct
B ☐ if 1 and 2 only are correct
C ☐ if 2 and 3 only are correct
D ☐ if 1 only is correct
E ☐ if 3 only is correct

Directions summarised				
A	**B**	**C**	**D**	**E**
1, 2, 3	1, 2 only	2, 3 only	1 only	3 only

Q36 Drugs that may cause jaundice include:

1 ☐ paracetamol
2 ☐ clomipramine
3 ☐ amoxicillin

Q37 Women who are taking a combined oral contraceptive are at an increased risk of:

1 ☐ deep-vein thrombosis during travel
2 ☐ fluid retention
3 ☐ chloasma

Q38 Diazepam:

1 ☐ produces amnesia
2 ☐ may produce an unnatural sleep pattern
3 ☐ causes CNS depression

Q39 Clinical features of hyperglycaemia include:

1 ☐ rapid pulse
2 ☐ hypertension
3 ☐ urinary retention

Q40 Hypoglycaemia in patients receiving antidiabetic treatment may be due to:

1 ☐ overeating
2 ☐ infection
3 ☐ unexpected exercise

Q41 Levocetirizine:

1 ☐ is not indicated for use in children aged under 1 year
2 ☐ adult dose is 5 mg daily
3 ☐ should be used with caution in epilepsy

Q42   Rabeprazole:

1   ☐ may mask symptoms of gastric cancer
2   ☐ may cause diarrhoea and abdominal pain as side-effects
3   ☐ requires three times daily administration

Q43   Loperamide:

1   ☐ slows intestinal motility
2   ☐ is presented in combination with atropine
3   ☐ should be recommended as a first-line treatment in melaena

Q44   Telithromycin:

1   ☐ is a derivative of erythromycin
2   ☐ is active against *Streptococcus pneumoniae*
3   ☐ should be used with caution in patients with cardiovascular disease

Q45   Ofloxacin:

1   ☐ has a broad spectrum of activity
2   ☐ is available as an ophthalmic preparation
3   ☐ does not have activity against *Pseudomonas aeruginosa*

Q46   Therapeutic equivalents to cefuroxime include:

1   ☐ cefaclor
2   ☐ ciprofloxacin
3   ☐ clindamycin

Q47   Mebendazole:

1   ☐ is indicated for roundworm
2   ☐ has vomiting as a common side-effect
3   ☐ brings about therapeutic action through reducing intestinal contents

Q48   Ibuprofen:

1   ❏ may be used for pyrexia in children
2   ❏ should be used with caution in patients with renal impairment
3   ❏ should not be used with paracetamol

Q49   Budesonide:

1   ❏ may be recommended for treatment of allergic rhinitis
2   ❏ is available as a nasal spray
3   ❏ should not be recommended to patients who have nasal polyps

Q50   Choline salicylate:

1   ❏ is used for mild oral lesions
2   ❏ may be used in paediatric patients over 4 months
3   ❏ may be applied every 30 minutes

Q51   Topical use of mepyramine:

1   ❏ may cause sensitisation
2   ❏ is only marginally effective
3   ❏ should be avoided in eczema

Q52   Mupirocin:

1   ❏ is a derivative of fusidic acid
2   ❏ may be used in the management of anaerobic infections
3   ❏ is indicated for *Staphylococcus aureus* infections

Q53 Povidone-iodine:

1 ☐ should be applied with care to broken skin
2 ☐ may be used in preoperative skin disinfection
3 ☐ is a phenol

Q54 The advice 'Do not transfer from this container' should be used for:

1 ☐ glyceryl trinitrate tablets
2 ☐ glyceryl trinitrate transdermal patch
3 ☐ isosorbide mononitrate tablets

Q55 Drugs that result in miosis include:

1 ☐ pilocarpine
2 ☐ carbachol
3 ☐ tropicamide

Q56 Gradual withdrawal of systemic corticosteroids is recommended:

1 ☐ whenever a dose of corticosteroids is administered
2 ☐ when treatment duration has been for 3 weeks or more
3 ☐ when repeat doses in the evening were given

Q57 Citalopram:

1 ☐ is not recommended in patients under 18 years
2 ☐ may cause nausea as a side-effect
3 ☐ should not be withdrawn abruptly

Q58 Methadone is:

1 ☐ an opioid agonist
2 ☐ addictive
3 ☐ only available as solid oral dosage forms

Q59 Tetracyclines that can be given on a once-daily dosing schedule include:

1 ☐ doxycycline
2 ☐ oxytetracycline
3 ☐ tetracycline

Q60 Cyanocobalamin:

1 ☐ may be found in multivitamin preparations
2 ☐ is vitamin B6
3 ☐ daily requirements are 100 mg

Questions 61–80

Directions: The following questions consist of a statement in the left-hand column followed by a second statement in the right-hand column. Decide whether the first statement is true or false. Decide whether the second statement is true or false. Then choose:

A ☐ if both statements are true and the second statement is a **correct explanation** of the first statement
B ☐ if both statements are true but the second statement **is NOT a correct explanation** of the first statement
C ☐ if the first statement is true but the second statement is false
D ☐ if the first statement is false but the second statement is true
E ☐ if both statements are false

Directions summarised			
	First statement	**Second statement**	
A	True	True	Second statement is a *correct* *explanation* of the first
B	True	True	Second statement is *NOT a correct* *explanation* of the first
C	True	False	
D	False	True	
E	False	False	

Q61 Patients taking carbimazole should be advised to report any sore throat. Carbimazole may cause a marked decrease in the number of granulocytes.

Q62 Methyldopa is a centrally-acting antihypertensive. Methyldopa may cause depression as a side-effect.

Q63 A diabetic patient with a history of angina is a candidate to receive simvastatin. Simvastatin may be used for secondary prevention of coronary events.

Q64 Diabetic patients are prone to ulceration in the feet. Diabetes may cause peripheral neuropathy.

Q65 Allergic conjunctivitis may be treated with levocabastine. Long-term use of levocabastine may cause glaucoma.

Q66 Nicotine replacement therapy may be administered as an inhalator. The inhalator is used when the urge to smoke occurs.

Q67 Tinea pedis has a wide distribution on the foot. Imidazole powder formulations are preferred to promote rapid healing.

Q68 Chronic back pain may indicate osteoporosis. In osteoporosis high calcium intake reduces the rate of bone loss.

Q69 Systemic therapy with ciprofloxacin may precipitate vulvovaginal candidiasis. Vulvovaginal candidiasis can only be treated with topical imidazole preparations.

Q70 In patients with renal disease, the use of citric acid and its salts in urinary tract infections is not associated with any sequelae. The use of these salts results in acidification of the urine.

Q71 Folinic acid is used to counteract methotrexate-induced mucositis. Methotrexate inhibits dihydrofolate reductase.

Q72 The temperature range required for a refrigerator is 2–8°C. A medicine indicated to be stored in a refrigerator may be stored in a deep freezer.

Q73 The term 'very soluble' means that the approximate volume of solvent in millilitres per gram of solute is less than 1. Only very soluble active ingredients are suitable for formulation in injectable dosage forms.

Q74 Semi-solid eye preparations contain one or more active ingredients dissolved or dispersed in a sterile base. None of the particles in a semi-solid eye preparation containing dispersed solid particles should have a maximum dimension greater than 90 µm.

Q75 Parenteral preparations may require the use of excipients. Excipients may be required to make the preparation isotonic with blood, to adjust the pH, to increase solubility, to prevent deterioration of the active ingredients or to provide adequate antimicrobial properties.

Q76 Syrups should be kept in well-closed containers and stored at temperatures not exceeding 30°C. Bacterial growth in syrups may occur in containers that are not well-closed and that are exposed to temperatures over 30°C.

Q77 Aromatic waters should not contain any traces of alcohol. Aromatic waters are saturated solutions of volatile oils or other aromatic substances in water.

Q78 Aciclovir tablets should be stored at a temperature not exceeding 25°C. Aciclovir tablets should be stored in the refrigerator.

Q79 Noradrenaline may be substituted for adrenaline in eye drops. Epinephrine is another name for adrenaline.

Q80 The term 'saline' is a code used on single-dose eye drop containers to indicate a 0.9% w/v solution of sodium chloride. Codes are approved for use on single-unit doses of eye drops where the individual container may be too small to bear all the appropriate labelling information.

Questions 81–85

These questions concern the following structure:

Q81 The structure represents a drug that is a (an):

A ☐ sympathomimetic
B ☐ antihistamine
C ☐ cholinergic agonist
D ☐ anticholinergic agent
E ☐ serotonin antagonist

Q82   An indication for use is:

A   ☐   asthma
B   ☐   migraine
C   ☐   nausea and vomiting
D   ☐   Parkinson's disease
E   ☐   motion sickness

Q83   The drug:

A   ☐   acts primarily on receptors in the peripheral system
B   ☐   presents a lag time with regards to onset of action
C   ☐   should be used with caution in hypertension
D   ☐   should be administered after food
E   ☐   induces diuresis

Q84   Adverse reactions to be expected include:

1   ☐   fine tremor
2   ☐   tachycardia
3   ☐   constipation

A   ☐   1, 2, 3
B   ☐   1, 2 only
C   ☐   2, 3 only
D   ☐   1 only
E   ☐   3 only

Q85   Essential features of the chemical structure for activity are:

1   ☐   amino group
2   ☐   aromatic ring
3   ☐   furan ring

A   ☐ 1, 2, 3
B   ☐ 1, 2 only
C   ☐ 2, 3 only
D   ☐ 1 only
E   ☐ 3 only

Questions 86–100

Directions: These questions involve prescriptions or patient requests. Read the prescription or patient request and select the best answer in each case.

Questions 86–87: Use the prescription below:

Patient's name   ....
Co-amoxiclav 625 mg tablets
bd   m 20
Doctor's signature   ....

Q86   Co-amoxiclav:

1   ☐ is a broad spectrum antibacterial agent
2   ☐ is less susceptible to inactivation by beta-lactamases
3   ☐ absorption is very limited

A   ☐ 1, 2, 3
B   ☐ 1, 2 only
C   ☐ 2, 3 only
D   ☐ 1 only
E   ☐ 3 only

Q87   This formulation:

1   ☐ consists of amoxicillin 625 mg
2   ☐ should not be administered at the same time as paracetamol
3   ☐ is given on a twice-daily dosing schedule

A   ☐ 1, 2, 3
B   ☐ 1, 2 only
C   ☐ 2, 3 only
D   ☐ 1 only
E   ☐ 3 only

Questions 88–92: Use the prescription below:

Patient's name   ....

Metronidazole tablets
400 mg tds   m 21

Doctor's signature   ....

Q88   Metronidazole could be:

1   ☐ used for anaerobic infections
2   ☐ used in combination with clarithromycin
3   ☐ used in animal bites

A   ☐ 1, 2, 3
B   ☐ 1, 2 only
C   ☐ 2, 3 only
D   ☐ 1 only
E   ☐ 3 only

Q89 Metronidazole is available as:

1 ☐ 200 mg tablets
2 ☐ 400 mg tablets
3 ☐ a suspension of 400 mg/5 mL

A ☐ 1, 2, 3
B ☐ 1, 2 only
C ☐ 2, 3 only
D ☐ 1 only
E ☐ 3 only

Q90 The patient should be advised:

1 ☐ to avoid alcoholic drink
2 ☐ to take with or after food
3 ☐ to avoid exposure to sunlight

A ☐ 1, 2, 3
B ☐ 1, 2 only
C ☐ 2, 3 only
D ☐ 1 only
E ☐ 3 only

Q91 Common side-effects that could occur include:

1 ☐ headache
2 ☐ unpleasant taste
3 ☐ rashes

A ☐ 1, 2, 3
B ☐ 1, 2 only
C ☐ 2, 3 only
D ☐ 1 only
E ☐ 3 only

Q92   Significant interactions could occur if metronidazole is administered concurrently with:

1   ☐ gliclazide
2   ☐ atenolol
3   ☐ warfarin

A   ☐ 1, 2, 3
B   ☐ 1, 2 only
C   ☐ 2, 3 only
D   ☐ 1 only
E   ☐ 3 only

Questions 93–96: Use the prescription below:

Patient's name   ....

Simvastatin 20 mg tablets
once daily   m 28

Doctor's signature   ....

Q93   Simvastatin:

1   ☐ lowers concentration of low density lipoprotein cholesterol
2   ☐ increases triglycerides
3   ☐ lowers concentration of high density lipoprotein cholesterol

A   ☐ 1, 2, 3
B   ☐ 1, 2 only
C   ☐ 2, 3 only
D   ☐ 1 only
E   ☐ 3 only

Q94 Simvastatin is indicated for secondary prevention of coronary and cardiovascular events in patients with:

1 ☐ angina
2 ☐ acute myocardial infarction
3 ☐ history of stroke

A ☐ 1, 2, 3
B ☐ 1, 2 only
C ☐ 2, 3 only
D ☐ 1 only
E ☐ 3 only

Q95 The patient should be advised:

1 ☐ to take the dose in the morning
2 ☐ that gastrointestinal side-effects may occur
3 ☐ to report muscle pain immediately

A ☐ 1, 2, 3
B ☐ 1, 2 only
C ☐ 2, 3 only
D ☐ 1 only
E ☐ 3 only

Q96 Before starting treatment with simvastatin the following tests should be carried out:

1 ☐ liver function tests
2 ☐ thyroid function tests
3 ☐ chest X-ray

A   ❑   1, 2, 3
B   ❑   1, 2 only
C   ❑   2, 3 only
D   ❑   1 only
E   ❑   3 only

Questions 97–100: Read the patient request.

> A patient who is on holiday presents with acute constipation. He has
> had the symptoms for the past 2 days.

For the following products, place your order of preference starting with 4 for the product that should be recommended as first choice and ending with 1 for the product that should be recommended as a last choice.

Q97   Lactulose

Q98   Liquid Paraffin

Q99   Magnesium Sulphate

Q100 Senna

Test 6

Answers

A1   D

In the pharmaceutical industry, the quality assurance department ensures that the plant's facilities and systems meet good manufacturing practice. The research and development department develops new drug entities and formulations. The analytical methods department works with the quality control department to develop and analyse raw materials, and to oversee quality during the manufacturing process and in the finished goods. The production department prepares the finished goods.

A2   B

Vitamin C, ascorbic acid, is a water-soluble vitamin that is required for the synthesis of collagen and intercellular material.

A3   E

Excessive alcohol consumption is not associated with dry mouth. Excessive consumption may cause memory impairment, vasodilation, dehydration, sensitivity to light, headache, increased salivation and damage to the gastric mucosa.

A4   C

Cathecol-O-methyltransferase (COMT) is an enzyme that is involved with the metabolic transformation of cathecholamines, including norepinephrine. It is available throughout the body. It causes methylation of catecholamines. Norepinephrine undergoes methylation mediated by COMT to normetanephrine.

A5 B

Carbidopa is a dopa-decarboxylase inhibitor that reduces the conversion of levodopa in the periphery before it reaches the brain. By administering levodopa with carbidopa, a lower dose of levodopa is required to achieve an effective brain-dopamine concentration.

A6 D

The resulting 2 L of a 1 in 1000 v/v solution contains 1 mL/1000 mL. Two millilitres are present in 2000 mL (2 L). In the 1 in 500 v/v solution, 1 mL is available in 500 mL, hence 2 mL are available in 1000 mL (500 × 2).

A7 B

In a 2% mixture, 2 g salicylic acid are present in 100 g. In 30 g, 0.6 g of salicylic acid are required (30 × 2/100).

A8 C

To prepare 100 g of the cream, 10 g of calamine are required. To prepare 60 g, 6 g are required (10 × 60/100).

A9 C

100 units are available in 1 mL. Twenty units are available in 0.2 mL (20/100).

A10 B

The daily dose of pivmecillinam to be administered is 240 mg (20 × 12). It is divided into three doses of 80 mg each.

A11   C

The daily dose required is 475 µg (95 × 5). The volume required is 1.58 mL (475/300).

A12   C

One milligram of disodium pamidronate is presented in 4.17 mL (250/60). To administer the solution at a rate not exceeding 1 mg/minute, not more than 4.17 mL/minute should be delivered. Delivering 4 mL/minute would result in the solution being administered within 62 minutes. Decreasing the amount of solution per minute results in an administration time greater than 90 minutes.

A13   B

Dopamine 800 µg is equivalent to 0.8 mg. The volume required is 0.02 mL (0.8/40).

A14   C

For a 0.9% saline solution, 0.9 g of sodium chloride are present in 100 mL. Thirty grams of sodium chloride would be present in 3333.3 mL (30 × 100/0.9), equivalent to 3.33 L.

A15   B

When 1 mg is dissolved in 500 mL, 100 mL of the solution contains 0.2 mg (100/500). This is equivalent to 0.0002 g in 100 mL. The percentage w/v is 0.0002%.

A16   B

Prochlorperazine is a phenothiazine and it acts as a dopamine antagonist. It is used in nausea and vomiting, vertigo and labyrinthine disorders, psychoses and anxiety.

A17   E

Lorazepam is a short-acting benzodiazepine that is indicated for short-term use in insomnia or anxiety. It enhances the activity of gamma-amino-butyric acid (GABA).

A18   C

Venlafaxine is a noradrenaline and serotonin re-uptake inhibitor (SNRI) that is used as an antidepressant agent in depressive illnesses. It may also be used in some anxiety disorders.

A19   A

Pergolide is a dopamine receptor agonist used in the management of parkinsonism.

A20   A

Orlistat is a lipase inhibitor used as an anti-obesity agent. Side-effects associated with its administration include oily leakage from the rectum, flatulence, faecal urgency, liquid or oily stools, faecal incontinence, abdominal distension and pain.

A21 C

Domperidone is a drug used in the management of nausea and vomiting. Rarely it causes gastrointestinal disturbances such as cramping and extrapyramidal effects.

A22 E

Sibutramine is a centrally acting appetite suppressant that inhibits re-uptake of noradrenaline and serotonin. Side-effects of sibutramine include constipation, dry mouth, nausea, taste disturbances, diarrhoea, vomiting, tachycardia, palpitations, hypertension, flushing, insomnia, lightheadedness, paraesthesia, headache, anxiety and depression.

A23 E

As sibutramine is a noradrenaline re-uptake inhibitor, it may cause hypertension as a side-effect.

A24 E

Furosemide is an anthranilic acid derivative with a sulfonamide moiety. It is used as a diuretic.

A25 E

Furosemide acts mainly at the ascending limb of the loop of Henle, inhibiting re-absorption of water and electrolytes.

A26   D

Spironolactone is a competitive antagonist of aldosterone, a mineralocorticoid agent that is responsible for enhancing re-absorption of sodium and secretion of potassium.

A27   D

As spironolactone has anti-androgenic activity, it may cause gynaecomastia as a side-effect. Side-effects of spironolactone also include gastrointestinal disturbances, impotence, menstrual irregularities and hyperkalaemia.

A28   E

Furosemide has a fast onset of action acting within 1 h of oral administration.

A29   D

Zinc oxide is a mild astringent that is used in preparations for haemorrhoids and in topical barrier preparations.

A30   B

Salicylic acid has keratolytic properties and is used in the management of hyperkeratotic conditions such as verrucas, corns and calluses.

A31   C

Aluminium salts, such as aluminium chloride hexahydrate, have antiperspirant effects when applied topically. It is used in preparations intended for the management of hyperhidrosis.

A32   C

Onchomycosis is a fungal nail infection that is difficult to treat. Treatment duration is long. Itraconazole, a triazole antifungal agent, presents fungicidal concentrations in the toenails resulting in clinical clearance of the infection.

A33   B

Ketoconazole, an imidazole antifungal agent, is available as a shampoo that is indicated for severe dandruff and seborrhoeic dermatitis affecting the scalp.

A34   D

Miconazole, an imidazole antifungal agent is available as gel for oral administration. It is not available in solid oral dosage forms.

A35   C

Heart failure has been reported after the systemic use of itraconazole. It should be used with caution in high-risk patients, such as those with a history of cardiac disease or who are taking negative inotropic drugs such as calcium-channel blockers.

A36   B

Paracetamol may cause jaundice when administered in excess of the recommended pharmacotherapeutic dose. Clomipramine may cause jaundice as a side-effect. Paracetamol and clomipramine are extensively metabolised in the liver. Paracetamol and clomipramine should be used with caution in patients with hepatic impairment. Amoxicillin is largely eliminated by the kidney.

A37 A

Travel, especially long-haul flights, is associated with an increased risk of deep-vein thrombosis. Women taking combined oral contraceptives (COCs) are at an increased risk of developing deep-vein thrombosis during travel. Fluid retention and chloasma are side-effects that are expected with COCs.

A38 A

Diazepam is a benzodiazepine that may produce amnesia as a side-effect. Common side-effects that may occur with benzodiazepines include drowsiness, sedation, muscle weakness and ataxia. These side-effects are due to the CNS depression caused by benzodiazepines. Benzodiazepines induce an unnatural sleep pattern because of rapid eye movement (REM) sleep suppression.

A39 D

Hyperglycaemia, which is raised blood glucose, produces osmotic diuresis. This results in a reduction in fluid volume, which leads to rapid pulse and hypotension. Another clinical feature of hyperglycaemia is polyuria, which is increased frequency of urination.

A40 E

Hypoglycaemia is a decreased blood glucose level. Its occurrence in patients receiving antidiabetic treatment may be due to excessive doses of insulin or oral antidiabetic agents and unexpected exercise. Overeating and infections may lead to hyperglycaemia.

A41 A

Levocetirizine is a non-sedating antihistamine that is used in adults and children over 6 years at a dose of 5 mg daily. It is not recommended for use in children under 1 year. As there have been occasional reports of convulsions with antihistamines, they should be used with caution in epilepsy.

A42   B

Rabeprazole is a proton pump inhibitor that may mask symptoms of gastric cancer because it may provide relief from symptoms of dyspepsia and gastro-oesophageal reflux caused by carcinoma. Side-effects of rabeprazole include gastrointestinal disturbances, such as diarrhoea and abdominal pain. The dosing frequency is normally once daily.

A43   D

Loperamide is an opioid drug used as an antimotility agent in the management of diarrhoea. Melaena, blood in stools, may be caused by a perforated ulcer or damaged inflamed areas in the gastrointestinal tract. It requires immediate referral.

A44   A

Telithromycin is a derivative of erythromycin that is used as an antibacterial agent and has a spectrum of activity similar to macrolides. It is also active against erythromycin-resistant *Streptococcus pneumoniae*. It has the potential to prolong the QT interval and should be used with caution in patients with cardiovascular disease.

A45   B

Ofloxacin is a quinolone with a broad spectrum of activity against Gram-negative aerobic bacteria including *Pseudomonas* species, Gram-positive aerobic bacteria and *Chlamydia*. It is available as an ophthalmic preparation and as a solution for administration in the ear.

A46   D

Cefuroxime and cefaclor are second-generation cephalosporins which are active against bacteria that are resistant to first-generation cephalosporins. Ciprofloxacin is a quinolone antibacterial agent whereas clindamycin is an antibacterial agent that is active against Gram-positive cocci and anaerobes.

A47   D

Mebendazole is a benzimidazole carbamate derivative that is indicated for infections with threadworms, roundworms, whipworm and hookworm. As it is poorly absorbed from the gastrointestinal tract, side-effects are rare and include abdominal pain and diarrhoea. Mebendazole acts by inhibiting or destroying cytoplasmic microtubules in the worm.

A48   B

Ibuprofen is a non-steroidal anti-inflammatory drug that can be used in children of over 7 kg body weight as an antipyretic and an analgesic. Ibuprofen may impair renal function and therefore it should be used with caution in patients with renal impairment. Paracetamol is a non-opioid analgesic with antipyretic and analgesic action with a different mode of action. They can be used concomitantly in reduction of fever or for analgesia.

A49   B

Budesonide is a corticosteroid available for nasal administration that may be used for prophylaxis and treatment of allergic and vasomotor rhinitis and for the management of nasal polyps. It is available as an aerosol spray, an aerosol inhaler and a turbohaler.

A50   B

Choline salicylate is available as a dental gel for use in mild oral and perioral lesions. It can be used in children over 4 months during teething. It is applied no more than every 3 h up to a maximum of six applications daily.

A51   A

Mepyramine is an antihistamine that is available as a topical dermatological preparation. It may cause hypersensitivity reactions and is only marginally effective. Topical use of mepyramine should be avoided in eczema because it may exacerbate the condition.

A52   E

Mupirocin is an antibacterial preparation that is effective for skin infections, particularly infections caused by Gram-positive organisms such as *Staphylococcus aureus*. It is not related to any other antibacterial agent.

A53   B

Povidone-iodine is an antiseptic agent based on iodine that may be used for pre and postoperative skin disinfection. It should be applied with caution to broken skin because it may cause systemic adverse effects, such as metabolic acidosis, hypernatraemia and renal function impairment.

A54   D

Glyceryl trinitrate tablets are unstable and patient should be advised not to transfer tablets from the container. Glyceryl trinitrate transdermal patches are packed individually in sealed packs. Isosorbide mononitrate tablets are not as unstable as glyceryl trinitrate.

A55 B

Miosis is the contraction of the pupil and it occurs as a result of administration to the eye of miotic preparations such as pilocarpine and carbachol that are used in raised intraocular pressure. Pilocarpine and carbachol are cholinergic agonists. Tropicamide is an antimuscarinic product that is used as a mydriatic for eye examination. Mydriasis is the dilation of the pupil, the opposite effect to miosis.

A56 C

When systemic corticosteroid therapy is given for a prolonged period, adrenal atrophy develops. Abrupt withdrawal of the steroid therapy may lead to acute adrenal insufficiency, hypotension or death. To prevent this, gradual withdrawal of systemic corticosteroids is recommended when treatment duration has been of 3 weeks or more and when repeat doses were given in the evening, because suppression of cortisol secretion is minimal if the dose is taken in the morning.

A57 A

Citalopram is a selective serotonin re-uptake inhibitor. Following reports that SSRIs may induce suicidal tendencies, they are not recommended for use in patients under 18 years. Common side-effects of SSRIs include gastrointestinal symptoms, such as nausea, vomiting, dyspepsia, abdominal pain, diarrhoea and constipation. Abrupt withdrawal of SSRIs is associated with a withdrawal syndrome that presents with headache, nausea, paraesthesia, dizziness and anxiety.

A58 B

Methadone is an opioid agonist that is used in the management of opioid dependence. It is itself self-addictive and prolonged use may cause dependence. However, withdrawal symptoms develop more slowly than with other opioid drugs. It is available as tablets and oral solution.

A59   D

Doxycycline is a tetracycline derivative that is very reliably absorbed and has a long half-life (12–24 h). It is given as a once-daily dose. Oxytetracyline and tetracycline have shorter half-lives (9 h) and they require multiple dosing daily.

A60   D

Cyanocobalamin is a cobalt-containing compound that is a vitamin B_{12} substance. Adult daily requirements for vitamin B_{12} are small, around 2 μg. Cyanocobalamin can be found in multivitamin preparations such as Forceval and Vivioptal.

A61   A

Carbimazole is an antithyroid drug that can cause bone marrow suppression leading to agranulocytosis, which is a decrease in the number of granulocytes. Signs of infection, such as sore throat, indicate bone marrow suppression.

A62   B

Methyldopa is an antihypertensive agent that has a central action resulting in a reduced sympathetic tone. This central activity leads to side-effects such as drowsiness, impaired concentration and memory, mild psychoses, depression and nightmares.

A63   A

Simvastatin is a lipid-regulating agent, which can be used for secondary prevention of coronary events in patients with coronary heart disease, peripheral artery disease and diabetes mellitus.

A64   A

Diabetes results in damage to nerves, which can lead to neuropathy and to impaired nervous conduction. Neuropathy in the peripheries, commonly the feet, can lead to injuries that subsequently develop into ulcerations. Diabetes causes peripheral vascular damage that predisposes the diabetic patient to infection and ulceration of the feet.

A65   C

Levocabastine is an antihistamine that may be used as a topical preparation in allergic conjunctivitis. Side-effects include local reactions (irritation, blurred vision, oedema, urticaria), dyspnoea and headache.

A66   B

Nicotine replacement therapy may be administered as chewing gum, inhalator, lozenges, nasal spray and patches. When the inhalator is used, the patient is advised to use it when the urge to smoke occurs.

A67   E

Tinea pedis is a fungal infection of the feet usually occurring in toe clefts. Sometimes the infection may spread and in severe cases the infection may extend to the toenails. Imidazole antifungals are used for the management of the condition as creams. Powder formulations are preferred for dusting footwear. Sometimes systemic administration of antifungal agents is required.

A68   B

Osteoporosis is characterised by pain. It occurs as a result of reduced bone mass, resulting in brittle bones commonly in the neck, vertebrae and wrists. Chronic back pain may indicate osteoporosis in the vertebrae. High calcium intake can be used in osteoporosis to reduce the rate of bone loss.

A69   C

Vulvovaginal candidiasis may occur with the systemic administration of ciprofloxacin because ciprofloxacin is a broad-spectrum antibacterial agent. Its use may result in superinfection with organisms such as *Candida* that are not susceptible to ciprofloxacin. Management of vulvovaginal candidiasis includes topical administration of imidazole antifungal agents and the systemic administration of fluconazole.

A70   E

Caution is recommended in the administration of citric acid and its salts to patients with renal disease as there may be metabolic consequences. Citric acid and its salts are used to alkalinise the urine and hence relieve the discomfort associated with cystitis.

A71   A

Methotrexate is an antimetabolite that inhibits dihydrofolate reductase, the enzyme involved in the reduction of folic acid to tetrahydrofolate. Folinic acid is used to counteract the decrease in tetrahydrofolate in normal cells. Folinic acid is given as rescue therapy to prevent side-effects caused by methotrexate therapy, namely mucositis and myelosuppression.

A72   C

The temperature required for a refrigerator is in the range 2–8°C and for a deep-freezer is –15°C. Items that are required to be stored in the refrigerator should not be kept in a deep freezer as this may compromise the product.

A73   C

According to the British Pharmacopoeia, 'very soluble' means that the approximate volume of solvent in millilitres per gram of solute is less than 1. Active ingredients of injectable dosage form preparations are not limited to very soluble materials. Suspensions are available for parenteral administration.

A74   B

Semi-solid eye preparations are products that are presented as sterile ointments, creams or gels intended for application to the conjunctiva. They consist of one or more active ingredients that are dissolved or dispersed in a sterile base. According to the British Pharmacopoiea, the maximum dimension of particles dispersed in semi-solid eye preparations should not exceed 90 μm.

A75   A

Parenteral preparations are sterile products intended for administration by injection, infusion or implantation. The preparations may require the use of excipients that should not interfere with the active ingredient or cause unwanted effects or local irritation. The excipients may be used to make the preparation isotonic with blood, to adjust the pH, to increase solubility, to prevent deterioration of the active ingredient or to provide adequate antimicrobial properties.

A76   A

Syrups are liquid preparations that are based on a concentrated solution of sucrose, other sugars or sweetening agents. Syrups should be kept in well-closed containers and stored at temperatures not exceeding 30°C, otherwise they are prone to bacterial growth.

A77   D

Aromatic waters are saturated solutions of volatile oils or other aromatic substances in water. According to the British Pharmacopoeia, aromatic waters are prepared using ethanol.

A78   C

Aciclovir tablets, which are indicated for the management of herpes simplex and varicella zoster infections, should be stored at room temperature, and no higher than 25°C. They should not be kept in a refrigerator.

A79   D

Adrenaline and noradrenaline are sympathomimetic agents. Adrenaline eye drops may be used in the management of open-angle glaucoma. Epinephrine is another name for adrenaline and norepinephrine is an alternate name for noradrenaline.

A80   A

The small size of single-dose containers for eye drops means that only an indication of the active ingredient and the strength of the preparation can be displayed. They are labelled using an approved code. The British Pharmacopoeia states codes for eye drops in single-dose containers. The code for sodium chloride is saline, indicating that the contents of the container are a 0.9% w/v solution.

A81   A

The structure represents a sympathomimetic amine, salbutamol, which has a substitution on the amino group, a hydroxyl group on the β carbon and a substituent on position 3 and 4 of the aromatic nucleus.

A82   A

Salbutamol, an adrenoceptor agonist, is used as a bronchodilator in asthma.

A83   C

As salbutamol is a sympathomimetic agent it should be used with caution in hypertension because it will activate the sympathetic nervous system, which in turn may result in increased blood pressure.

A84   B

Side-effects that may occur with salbutamol include fine tremor, nervous tension, headache, muscle cramps and tachycardia.

A85   B

The chemical structure of sympathomimetic agents is based on an aromatic ring that is separated by two carbon atoms from an amino group. Substitutions on the structure result in the various sympathomimetic drugs.

A86 B

Co-amoxiclav consists of amoxicillin, a broad spectrum penicillin, and clavu-lanic acid. Clavulanic acid is a product that lacks antibacterial properties. It inactivates beta-lactamases, the enzymes that destroy the beta-lactam ring and result in inactivation of the penicillin. Amoxicillin is more rapidly and more completely absorbed compared with ampicillin, which is moderately well absorbed from the gastrointestinal tract. The presence of food in the stomach does not appear to interfere with the amount of amoxicillin absorbed.

A87 E

Co-amoxiclav 625 mg tablets contain amoxicillin 500 mg and clavulanic acid 125 mg. The drug is given on a twice daily dosing schedule. Patient should be advised to take the drug as prescribed at regular intervals and to complete the course of treatment.

A88 A

Metronidazole is an anti-infective agent that can be used against anaerobic bacteria and protozoa. It can be used in combination with clarithromycin where necessary. It is combined with clarithromycin in triple therapy for *Helicobacter pylori* eradication. Animal bites may be associated with infections caused by anaerobic bacteria.

A89 B

Metronidazole is available for oral administration as tablets of 200 mg and 400 mg and as a suspension of 200 mg/5 mL.

A90 B

The patient should be advised to avoid alcoholic drink, to take the drug at regular intervals and to complete the course prescribed, to take the tablets with or after food, and to swallow them whole with plenty of water. When patients taking metronidazole consume alcohol, a disulfiram-like reaction may occur.

A91 A

Side-effects that may occur with metronidazole include nausea, vomiting, unpleasant taste, furred tongue, gastrointestinal disturbances, rashes and headache.

A92 E

A significant clinical interaction can occur between metronidazole and warfarin. It is advisable to avoid concomitant use because metronidazole enhances the anticoagulant effect of warfarin.

A93 D

Simvastatin is a lipid-regulating drug that results in a lowering of the concentration of low-density lipoprotein cholesterol that is associated with hyperlipidaemia. It may result in lowering of triglycerides but statins are less effective in this than the fibrates.

A94 A

Statins are used for the secondary prevention of coronary and cardiovascular events in patients with a history of angina, acute myocardial infarction and history of stroke.

A95   C

Patient should be advised to take the tablet at night to counteract the nocturnal increase in cholesterol synthesis. Side-effects of simvastatin include gastrointestinal effects such as abdominal pain, flatulence, constipation or diarrhoea, nausea and vomiting. As simvastatin can cause myopathy that could lead to rhabdomyolysis, the patient should be advised to report muscle pain, tenderness or weakness immediately.

A96   B

Statins should be used with caution in patients with a history of liver disease, and hypothyroidism should be managed adequately before starting treatment with a statin. It is recommended that liver function tests and thyroid function tests are performed before starting treatment with simvastatin.

A97–A100

A laxative that has a rapid action is required to provide immediate relief. A stimulant laxative such as senna may be recommended for the short term. Lactulose, an osmotic laxative, has a delayed onset. It may take up to 48 h to act and therefore it is not recommended as a single agent for the management of an acute phase. Magnesium sulphate is an osmotic laxative that brings about rapid bowel evacuation. This may result in electrolyte imbalance and its use as a laxative is reserved for when complete bowel evacuation is necessary, such as before a surgical intervention. Owing to the disadvantages associated with the use of liquid paraffin, its use is not supported. It may cause anal irritation, lipid pneumonia and interference with the absorption of fat-soluble vitamins.

A97 3

A98 1

A99 2

A100 4

Section 3

Sequential questions

Test 7

Questions

Directions: For the following questions, the five answers have a different probability of being correct. Indicate the sequential order of the five answers. (Scoring may be developed to reflect a different weighting for each answer.)

Q1 Arrange the following molecules according to their molecular weight. Start with 1 for the molecule with the lowest molecular weight up to 5 for the molecule with the highest molecular weight:

A ☐ glucose
B ☐ sucrose
C ☐ glycerine
D ☐ aluminium chloride
E ☐ sodium chloride

Q2 Arrange the following reactions according to their probability of happening spontaneously in the aspirin molecule, in a neutral medium under normal temperature and pressure conditions. Start with 1 for the reaction with the lowest probability up to 5 for the reaction with the highest probability:

A ☐ hydrolysis of ethanoate group
B ☐ partial reduction of the aromatic ring
C ☐ oxidation of the aromatic ring
D ☐ racemisation
E ☐ formation of intramolecular H-bonding

Q3 Different classes of medicines are used in the management of hypertension. Arrange the following classes of antihypertensive agents, starting with the one that has been longest on the market:

A ☐ sympatholytics
B ☐ calcium-channel blockers
C ☐ angiotensin-II receptor antagonists
D ☐ ACE inhibitors
E ☐ diuretics

Q4 Arrange the following classes of drugs used for the treatment of hypertension according to their selling price, starting with the least expensive:

A ☐ centrally acting antihypertensive drugs
B ☐ calcium-channel blockers
C ☐ angiotensin-II receptor antagonists
D ☐ beta-adrenoceptor blocking drugs
E ☐ diuretics

Q5 The following statements list more than one property of the compounds A (clonidine) and B (imipramine); all or none may be correct. Arrange the statements according to their correctness. Start with 1 for the least correct answer up to 5 for the most correct answer:

A ☐ structure A: bicyclic, neutral, insoluble in water
B ☐ structure A: basic, soluble in HCl 2N
C ☐ structure A: acid, soluble in NaOH 2N
D ☐ structure B: tricyclic, basic, soluble in HCl 2N
E ☐ structure B: bicyclic, acid, soluble in water

Q6 The following statements interpret the meaning of 'generic substitution' and 'therapeutic substitution' to different levels of correctness. Arrange the statements, starting with 1 for the least likely answer up to 5 for the most likely:

A ☐ both terms refer to the substitution of a drug
B ☐ both terms refer to the substitution of a drug with another generic product
C ☐ the terms are correlated with the professional experience of the nurse present in the hospital during the drug dispensing
D ☐ the terms refer to the substitution with a generic drug and any other suitable drug respectively
E ☐ the terms are exclusively correlated with the change of dosage

Q7 All factors being equal, arrange the bioavailability of the following formulations. Start with the formulation with the least degree of bioavailability:

A ☐ suspension
B ☐ capsule
C ☐ emulsion
D ☐ tablets
E ☐ solutions

Q8 The following statements list properties of the compound nalorphine. Arrange the statements, starting with 1 for the least likely answer up to 5 for the most likely. Nalorphine:

A ☐ induces analgesia but not euphoria
B ☐ binds mainly to the μ, δ and κ receptors of opiates
C ☐ has a pharmacological action similar to that of encephaline
D ☐ has a pharmacological action similar to that of naloxone
E ☐ does not belong to the opioid class of drugs

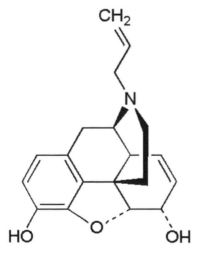

Q9 Arrange in ascending order the following salts according to the pH when the salts are dissolved in water at the same concentrations. Start with the lowest pH as 1 and the highest pH as 5:

A ☐ morphine hydrochloride
B ☐ sodium benzoate
C ☐ sodium phenate
D ☐ potassium chloride
E ☐ sodium salicylate

Q10 The narcotic analgesics have a structure correlated with the pentacyclic structure of morphine. Arrange the following cycles found in the morphine formula. Start with 1 for the cycle not found in the largest number of narcotic analgesics up to 5 for the one found in most narcotic analgesics:

A ☐ furan
B ☐ benzene
C ☐ cyclohexane
D ☐ cyclohexene
E ☐ piperidine

Test 7

Answers

A1

The molecular weight is the sum of the atomic weights of all the atoms in the molecule. Glucose is a monosaccharide with six carbon atoms and six oxygen atoms whereas sucrose is a disaccharide that has 12 carbon atoms and 11 oxygen atoms. Glycerine is a polyalcohol with three carbon atoms and three oxygen atoms. The number of hydrogen atoms can be ignored in these three molecules, because hydrogen has a molecular weight of 1 and therefore it is not a determining factor. Consequently the molecular weight in decreasing order is sucrose, glucose, glycerine. Aluminium is a trivalent atom and its chloride salt has three chlorine atoms. Sodium is a monovalent atom and its chloride salt has one chlorine atom. There are thus two series of compounds with molecular weights in descending order: sucrose, glucose, glycerine and aluminium chloride, sodium chloride. Comparing the lowest molecular weight of the compounds in the first series with the highest molecular weight of the compounds in the second series, glycerine has three atoms of carbon and three atoms of oxygen, whereas aluminium chloride has one atom of aluminium and three atoms of chlorine. Each pair of carbon–oxygen atoms has a weight of 28 whereas each chlorine atom has a weight of 35. Aluminium has an atomic weight of 27 and the three atoms of chlorine weigh 105. Hence aluminium chloride lies between glycerine and glucose. When comparing sodium chloride and glycerine, the three pairs of carbon and oxygen atoms in glycerine have a combined weight of 84 (28 × 3) whereas sodium chloride has a combined weight of 23 (atomic weight of sodium) plus 35 (atomic weight of chlorine) giving a molecular weight of 58.

A   ☐ 4
B   ☐ 5
C   ☐ 2
D   ☐ 3
E   ☐ 1

A2

The chemical structure of aspirin (acetylsalicylic acid) consists of an aromatic ring, a carboxyl moiety and a phenolic hydroxide esterified with acetic acid. Racemization of aspirin is impossible because it requires a chiral molecule. Aspirin does not have an asymmetric carbon atom and therefore is not a chiral molecule. The aromatic ring is very stable and hence it is not very reactive. Its total or partial reduction can occur by hydrogenation only in the presence of the appropriate catalysts and under high pressure. The oxidization of the aromatic ring is very difficult but, under certain conditions (for example, in the presence of free oxygen radicals), such a reaction can occur under mild conditions as, for example, when aspirin is used therapeutically and interacts within the arachidonic acid cascade *in vivo*. If aspirin is kept in a damp place, partial hydrolysis of the molecule may occur even at room temperature. Intramolecular hydrogen bonding is easily formed in aspirin. The planar structure of the acetylsalicylic acid molecule allows interaction between the hydrogen atom of the carboxyl group and the phenolic oxygen of the ester group. The resulting six-cyclic structure, which forms without energy, is quite stable.

A ☐ 4
B ☐ 2
C ☐ 3
D ☐ 1
E ☐ 5

A3

Among the classes listed, diuretics (thiazides, 1950) were the earliest group to be released on the market followed by the sympatholytics (beta-adreno-ceptor blocking agents such as propranolol, 1960), angiotensin-converting enzyme inhibitors such as captopril (1976), calcium-channel blockers such as nifedipine (1980) and angiotensin II receptor antagonists such as losartan (1990).

A ❑ 2
B ❑ 4
C ❑ 5
D ❑ 3
E ❑ 1

A4

The cost of antihypertensive drugs varies according to the time of their introduction to the market. The cost of medicines is affected by the validity of the
patent rights of each drug entity and by the introduction of the corresponding
generic pharmaceutical products on the market. The sequence of the cost of
the medicines in ascending order is: diuretics (thiazides such as bendroflumethiazide), centrally acting antihypertensive drugs such as methyldopa and
clonidine, beta-adrenoceptor blocking agents such as atenolol, calcium-
channel blockers such as nifedipine and angiotensin-II antagonists such as
losartan.

A ❑ 2
B ❑ 4
C ❑ 5
D ❑ 3
E ❑ 1

A5

The term 'polycyclic' applies to molecules that consist of partial cyclic structures, which together form one extensive cyclic system. Structure A has two
isolated cycles and hence cannot be termed polycyclic whereas structure B
has three condensed cycles and is a polycyclic, specifically a tricyclic structure. The acidic or basic characteristics of a molecule are related to the
presence of acid functions (most commonly carboxylic or sulphonic groups) or
basic functions (for example amino groups linked to aliphatic or aromatic

residues) respectively. Acidic or basic substances, even when insoluble in water, dissolve quickly in alkaline or acidic solutions respectively; this behaviour is due to the formation of ionic substances (salts) that are formed under these conditions. In fact, organic molecules are soluble in water when they have a low molecular weight, when they can be ionized (salts) or when the molecule has an adequate number of polar groups in relation to the molecular structure. Both clonidine and imipramine are basic substances owing to the saturated imidazole group in clonidine and the tertiary amine group in imipramine. The nitrogen atom bonded to the benzene ring also contributes to the basic property. Considering the correct and incorrect characteristics given in each statement, the answer is:

A ☐ 3
B ☐ 4
C ☐ 2
D ☐ 5
E ☐ 1

A6

The term 'generic drug' refers to drugs where patent rights of the active ingredient have expired and where the name of the product is identical to the generic (not proprietary) name of the active ingredient. The term 'off-patent drugs' is a vast classification because, besides the 'generic drugs', it includes drugs where patent rights have expired but that retain a proprietary name designated by the manufacturing company, instead of being known by the generic name of the active ingredients. In some countries the pharmacist may undertake generic substitution where the prescribed generic drug can be substituted with another generic drug presenting the same active ingredient. Some countries restrict generic substitution to when the patent rights have expired on the prescribed drug and the replacement product is less expensive. In countries where legislation allows therapeutic substitution, the pharmacist may change the medicine for another that has the same pharmacological action and therapeutic effect as the prescribed product. Both answers C and E do not fulfil these explanations and moreover, answer C does not relate to either of the terms considered. Answers going from B, D to A are gradually more realistic: answer B explains the term generic substitution but does not include therapeutic substitution; answer D states that the substituted drug has to be a generic to explain the term generic substitution and has to be any other drug to explain the term therapeutic substitution. Both the terms generic and therapeutic substitution refer to the substitution of a drug, as correctly stated in answer A.

A   ❑ 5
B   ❑ 3
C   ❑ 1
D   ❑ 4
E   ❑ 2

A7

Bioavailability may be measured by determining the concentration of active ingredient in plasma. The pharmaceutical formulations presented in the question are intended for oral drug administration. With this route of administration, the bioavailability of the drug reaches its maximum when the active ingredient is presented in a formulation that allows rapid dissolution into the biological fluids. Therefore, bioavailability is at its maximum with solutions followed by suspensions and emulsions, the latter consisting of solid or oily particles of small dimensions dispersed in a liquid formulation. Bioavailability is lower for the solid oral dosage forms. With capsules, the granules have to be released from the shell before dissolution and with tablets disintegration followed by dissolution has to take place for the release of the active ingredient. Disintegration is in most cases a longer process than release from a capsule shell.

A   ❑ 4
B   ❑ 2
C   ❑ 3
D   ❑ 1
E   ❑ 5

A8

Nalorphine and naloxone are structurally related to morphine and in fact are opioid drugs. When they bind to the analgesic receptor, they do not elicit the same response, owing to steric factors. Naloxone is an antagonist whereas nalorphine is a partial agonist. Nalorphine has a pharmacological action similar to encephaline in that both act on the κ (kappa) receptor, producing analgesia and sedation. Nalorphine binds with difficulty at the μ (mu) receptor and, in contrast to encephaline, nalorphine acts as an antagonist. Owing to this characteristic nalorphine induces analgesia with no euphoria.

Nalorphine   Naloxone

A ☐ 5
B ☐ 3
C ☐ 4
D ☐ 2
E ☐ 1

A9

Salts are formed through a reaction between an acid and a base. When the base and the acid are both strong (acids and mineral bases), the salt obtained when they are dissolved in water does not have the feature of hydrolysis and so the aqueous solution has a pH of 7. When salts formed from weak acids and strong bases (or weak bases and strong acids) are dissolved in water they hydrolyse. Hydrolysis produces solutions with a pH lower than 7 when the acid is stronger than the base and with a pH higher than 7 when the base is stronger than the acid. The numerical value of the positive or negative divergence from the value 7 correlates with the different strength of the acids or the bases, indicated by the corresponding values of pK_a and pK_b (the higher the value, the lower the strength of the acid). Morphine hydrochloride is formed from a strong mineral acid and a weak organic base. When dissolved in water, acid hydrolysis occurs and the resulting solution has a pH value lower than 7. In the case of potassium chloride, formed by a reaction between a strong acid and a strong base, hydrolysis does not occur, which means that the pH of the solution remains at 7. The other three salts mentioned are formed by a reaction between sodium hydroxide and organic acids (that is between a strong base and a weak acid). When dissolved in water they give a basic solution with a pH as high as the pK_a of the acid present in the salt. Of the two carboxylic acids discussed, salicylic acid ($pK_a = 3$) is stronger than benzoic acid ($pK_a = 4.2$) because of the phenolic hydroxyl group at the ortho position. Such a difference of pK_a is the reason for the lower value of pH in the aqueous solution of sodium salicylate in contrast to that of sodium benzoate. The low acidity of phenolic hydroxyl ($pK_a = 10$) brings about the strong alkaline hydrolysis of sodium phenate, the solution of which has a pH of 10.

A   ☐   1
B   ☐   4
C   ☐   5
D   ☐   2
E   ☐   3

A10

Among the natural and synthetic compounds having an analgesic–narcotic effect, most structures have the benzene ring, which is present in morphine. Such a group is therefore required for the compound to have an analgesic effect. The piperidine ring is present in all known narcotic analgesic structures, with the exception of two synthetic compounds (methadone and propoxyphene). These have an amino group in an open carbon chain, which on the receptor behaves in a similar way to the piperidine ring. The cyclohexane ring is not found in the analgesics meperidine, methadone and pethidine. The cyclohexene ring is not found in the analgesics phenazocine, meperidine, methadone, pentazocine, pethidine and propoxyphene. The furan ring is found only in the natural alkaloids of opium but not in most analgesics, for example, phenazocine, meperidine, methadone, pentazocine, pethidine and propoxyphene.

A ☐ 1
B ☐ 5
C ☐ 3
D ☐ 2
E ☐ 4

Explanatory notes

Open-book section

Test 1 questions are used as examples for general comments.

Questions 1–10

The 10 questions follow a pattern where each of the questions or incomplete statements are followed by five suggested answers; the candidate has to select the best answer in every case. Although you are asked to select the 'best' answer in these questions, quite often there is only one good answer.

(This differs from the newly introduced type of question where you are asked to list the answers in order of merit in their suitability ranking, from the least probable answer to the most probable answer (*see* Test 7). These types of questions will be dealt with at a later stage. They are considered to be of a more difficult nature.)

The following are some of the areas dealt with in Q1–10:

1   route of drug administration
2   alternative drugs for a presented condition
3   properties and indications of a particular drug
4   characteristics of diseases
5   triggering factors for a condition
6   constituents of a proprietary preparation
7   good pharmacy practice.

The answers to two questions out of these 10, namely Q6 and Q10, which were commonly answered incorrectly, were not to be found in texts such as the *British National Formulary* (BNF). The answer to Q6 could easily be deduced by referring to the reference book *Minor Illness or Major Disease* using an exclusion exercise to determine that it is sleep that does not trigger migraine.

The registration examination gives the right to the pharmacist to belong to an august body of professionals who, in addition to knowledge and skills, possess other attributes needed for good professional practice. One such attribute is a knowledge of the governance of pharmacy locally and internationally, especially in relation to good pharmacy practice. Q10 seeks to establish this attribute in the candidate. The answer to Q10, which deals with the function of professional organisations, can be found in one of the reference books recommended, namely *Validation Instruments for Community Pharmacists*.

The fact that a pharmacist is a fully fledged professional cannot be overemphasised. A number of questions to ascertain the candidates' appreciation of this are sometimes included in pre-registration examinations. For example, examination boards for various professions include questions related to historical facts concerning the particular profession.

Questions 11–34

These questions are an exercise in matching a drug with a feature characteristic of that drug. The matching involves drug effects, dosing, cautionary labels, dosage forms, proprietary names and physical characteristics.

Q11–13 and Q31–34 were more common in past papers. These types of questions are comparatively easy and they are only meant to familiarise the reader with MCQs and with using reference books such as the BNF efficiently and effectively. In later tests such simple questions are eliminated. It is important to check even in these straightforward cases that you do not make mistakes; remember that marks lost on easy questions are the same as those lost on harder ones.

Q14–20: These seven questions relate to the identification of various properties and effects of drugs. It has been noted that even pharmacists who make regular reference to formularies sometimes miss the wealth of information available in the appendices. Such was the case in those candidates who answered question 19 incorrectly; the answer could easily be found by referring to BNF Appendix 4, dedicated totally to pregnancy.

Formularies such as the BNF often carry appendices dedicated to important topics such as interactions, liver disease, renal impairment, pregnancy, intravenous additives, borderline substances, wound management products and elastic hosiery, and cautionary and advisory labels for dispensed medicines. The astute candidate will be familiar with these appendices by routinely referring to them during the preregistration practice. Many other countries have resource books similar to the BNF, such as the *Prontuario Terapeutico* published by the Ministry of Health in Portugal and the *Physicians' Desk Reference* in the United States of America.

Q24 is one of the few questions that fewer than half of the candidates got right. In such cases, although the BNF clearly indicates the correct answer, the examiners may decide to withdraw the question from the examination and adjust the candidates' marks accordingly. This question has been included in this publication to make it as close a simulation to an actual examination as possible. Following each sitting of the examination, many examination boards scrutinise the marked sheets and collect statistical information. Examiners review the questions with emphasis on the number of candidates who get each question right and any anomalies related to the candidates' performance are picked up. Invariably, following this exercise, there will be the odd question where one could argue that more than one correct answer was possible. Such a question may be removed from the marking pool. In addition, a check is carried out to ensure that such a deletion causes no candidate to move from pass to fail for this reason only. Q24 might perhaps fall in this category. This point is made to emphasise that in the case of those examination boards that do not carry a negative marking system for wrong answers, it is important that candidates should answer all questions to the best of their ability, keeping strictly to the instructions as to how to answer the questions, whether or not they feel that the question may contain a mistake.

In the case of Q24, because the candidate is only allowed to select one label, you should choose the one that is most relevant. In the case of an open-book test such as this, the label indicated by the BNF would be the best choice. On the very rare occasions when a question is deemed to be truly ambiguous, the examination board has the power to apply the necessary remedy. The student has no obligation or right to indicate examination errors on the paper. Such indication or marking on the paper may invalidate the candidate's paper especially in those cases where an index number is used and the candidates' identities are hidden from the examiners or administrators. The candidate should assume that there are no errors in the examination paper because the rigour of the examination setting process has shown that this is so, except in rare instances. This will be taken into consideration during the marking validation and the completeness of the quality assurance of the examination is always ensured.

Q31–34: The setting of questions that relate to the colour and strength of a particular tablet is sometimes questioned because good practice demands that pharmacists should not rely solely upon the colour of a product to identify the drug. This would be a hugely risky strategy and should not be encouraged. However the questions are meant to test the ability of candidates to use texts such as the BNF in day-to-day practice. In particular it reminds pharmacists not to rely on memory but to verify with a text. Tablets of the same medicine vary in colour from one country to another. In this case you should practise the questions by making the necessary changes according to the particular country. Notwithstanding the simplicity of such questions there were candidates who gave the wrong answer.

Questions 35–60

These questions are slightly harder than the previous 34 questions. In the first instance the question may be marked wrong if you do not know the correct answer to any of the three statements. Second, although you can always verify a correct statement in the reference books, there is no easy way to check that a statement is not correct. This is where the judicious use of the references available in an open-book examination is important. You have to be careful not to spend precious time looking for data that does not exist in any of the reference books because the statement is not right. The rule of thumb, which is not infallible, is that if you do not know from your own knowledge base that a statement is true, and the statement does not appear in the reference texts, you should assume that it is a false statement.

In all cases it is very important to read the question very carefully. Q37 is a case in point. The key word in this question is *hazardous*. Certain interactions mentioned in this question may occur but are not potentially hazardous. The BNF again serves as a good reference to identify those interactions that are classified as potentially hazardous.

In a pharmacy examination, candidates expect to be examined mainly on drugs. They are sometimes taken unawares when they meet with questions such as Q40, which concerns a condition without any reference to a drug. In Q40 the term used was capsulitis. It could have been another condition. Going through the recommended reference books such as *Minor Illness or Major Disease?* and *Handbook of Pharmacy Health Care* helps to give an indication of some of the conditions that a pharmacist is expected to be familiar with.

Questions 61–80

These questions require more thinking than looking carefully at straightforward factual material. The questions consist of groups of two statements and you have to decide whether each statement is true or false, then, if both statements are correct, if the second statement is a correct explanation of the first. A question may therefore require three decisions. In this case a mistake in one of the decisions would mean gaining no marks.

Some examination boards have a negative marking system (e.g. deducting a point for questions answered wrongly and no deduction for unattempted questions). The system adopted often depends on the type of questions set. Simple true and false questions usually carry a deduction for wrong questions, to compensate for the marks gained only through guesswork and chance (negative marking). These often carry a loss of a half to a full point. No simple true-or-false questions are set in the tests presented in this book. The decision whether to apply a negative marking system often also depends on the percentage pass mark required for a particular examination. At present, for example, the examinations set for registration by the Royal Pharmaceutical Society of Great Britain (RPSGB) require 70% minimum as a pass mark and carry no negative marking.

Some boards have a negative marking system for certain parts of the examination and no negative marking for other parts. For example, in Test 1 Q1–60 could be marked with a negative marking for wrong answers whereas Q61–80 would carry no negative marking. You should therefore carefully read the instructions for the examination board of the state or country for which you are sitting. You should familiarise yourself with the particular examination system in good time, before starting to prepare for the examination.

In addition to the examination syllabus for preregistration training for the specific year, the RPSGB publishes registration examination guidance notes, a set of examination regulations and registration examination sample papers for Part I (Closed-Book) and for Part II (Open-Book and Calculations). These documents are available on the RPSGB website. You should make sure that you have up-to-date documents pertaining to the examination sittings that you intend to take. A lack of thorough familiarisation often results in a significant loss of marks in questions like Q61–80.

In Q61–80 when both statements are correct, candidates often go wrong in deciding whether the second statement is a true and correct explanation of the first. Q61 and Q62 both contained two true statements each but the second statement does not explain the first. It is strange how many candidates opt that the second statement explains the first, even when this answer is clearly illogical even from a simple syntax analysis. Q70 is an example that indicates the tendency for students to 'hear alarm bells' when they read the word 'toxicity'. They seem to have a propensity for classifying a statement as true when it mentions that a substance produces toxicity, without giving it careful thought. Most pharmacy students are well aware that not all drugs that enter milk are toxic to infants. Yet candidates confuse 'are' with 'may be'. This is a common mistake, as shown by the 87% who got Q70 wrong.

Q80 is an example where students mix up terms such as 'motion sickness' and 'vertigo' and hence misidentify an indication for a drug. There is a tendency for candidates in an open-book examination to try to rely solely on finding the answer to the question in the references allowed in the examination. An interaction and assimilation of practice experience and the use of reference texts is essential in open-book examinations. It is clear that those many candidates who decided that betahistine is indicated for motion sickness in Q80 had not recalled what happens in real pharmacy practice. Who has witnessed the dispensing of betahistine for motion sickness in a community pharmacy? Lack of corroboration of theory with practice is often found to be a characteristic of those who fail registration examinations.

Questions 81–100

These questions deal with prescriptions and patients' requests. Although the questions regarding prescription preparations were commonly answered correctly, those dealing with patients' requests for non-prescription preparations and those that called for specific instructions were more often answered incorrectly. Pay special attention to which preparations, especially non-prescription preparations, are recommended for use in children, and to those that are not. A number of preparations, including some available in liquid form, are not suitable for children. Some candidates are confused by the fact that the dosage form is a liquid and assume that it is appropriate for children but certain syrups, such as Vicks Medinite, are not recommended for a 5 year old.

Relate the question to 'real life' situations. This advice cannot be overemphasised for all questions, but especially for Q81–100. Place yourself in a real pharmacy at that point in time. What would you do in such a case? The answer you would give in a real situation has a good chance of being the correct one in the examination.

Closed-book section

Test 4–6 questions are used as examples for general comments.

One of the most important sections in a closed-book examination in pharmacy is the one dealing with mathematics, better known as pharmaceutical calculations. This is dealt with in detail below under the heading 'Mathematical Thinking'.

A number of examination boards specify that the calculations section of the examination must be passed in a non-compensatory manner. The registration examination guidance notes of the Royal Pharmaceutical Society of Great Britain (RPSGB) published for the preregistration training 2004/05, in the section describing how the examination is marked, state that to pass the examination you must achieve 70% overall, that is, across all questions, *and* you must achieve 70% in the section of 20 calculation-style questions. If you do not achieve 70% overall but 70% in the calculation section, you have to resit the examination. This also means that notwithstanding how excellently you perform in all other parts of the examination, failure to pass the mathematical part leads to a failure in the whole examination. For this reason many candidates are in a state of panic when tackling this section. A few hints on how to approach the mathematical part are therefore in order.

Mathematical thinking

This section, which is covered in the closed-book examination in Test 4 Q8–11, Test 5 Q6–12 and Test 6 Q6–15, considers the topic in greater detail.

In realising the importance given to pharmaceutical calculations, you should keep in mind that a wrong calculation in real life can result in a fatal incident, which should be avoided under all circumstances. As is to be expected, the pharmacist is very often the person responsible for making correct pharmaceutical calculations.

The problem that candidates have in performing satisfactorily in the calculations section is often the result of an old-fashioned approach to teaching mathematics. The subject was often undertaken as a drill in repetitive manipulation of numbers according to some magic formula. Adopt a different approach for doing successful calculations throughout your career. The *raison d'être* of studying pharmaceutical calculations in pharmacy education should be the need to solve practical, everyday pharmaceutical problems; students should train to use mathematics in other areas of learning besides purely pharmaceutical calculations. By reasoning logically, an answer to a problem that results in giving a patient a 1 kg tablet should immediately indicate that the answer is incorrect, however certain you are that you have applied the appropriate formula.

The basic reasoning behind all calculations should reflect mathematical thinking. It is of little use learning several formulas to apply during an examination, if you cannot get the correct answer or identify a clear error. Completing whole sets of exercises in a repetitive manner is fruitless effort if you do not know how to handle a situation that is unfamiliar, or how to carry out a task that is presented in a practical rather than in a theoretical format.

You are advised to develop a three-pronged approach to mathematical practice, namely, reasoning, communicating and solving problems. Reasoning mathematically involves students in searching for patterns and relationships within their mathematical work, moving from textbook examples to practical examples during their preregistration practice and considering whether the answer makes logical sense. Seek opportunities to talk and reason mathematically rather than to rely solely on the recommendation of, say, a particular dosage regimen for children as stated on the package insert or in a written text. Does the recommended dose match the dose worked out by you?

During your preregistration practice, you must learn to communicate mathematically. Mathematical language should be used correctly in all day-to-day communications. For example, a liquid preparation should be described as 250 mg/5 mL and not just 250 mg. The proper units must accompany all numbers.

Calculating correctly is useless if the result is then written incorrectly, for example, by placing a decimal point in the wrong position. Mathematical terminology and language must be correct at all times. For instance, percentages should always be followed by w/w, w/v, v/w or v/v.

The third step should be the solving of problems in a variety of contexts. Pharmacists must be numerate, and avoidance of use of calculators for minor needs should be encouraged. In a community pharmacy a bill can be mentally approximated and then the result matched with the till or cashpoint as an exercise in mental arithmetic.

Such exercises, even if not strictly of a pharmaceutical nature, get the mind working with numbers and can serve you well, especially in those board examinations where the use of a calculator is not permitted. The registration examination guidance notes of the RPSGB for the preregistration training 2004/05 state that in the examination the candidate will be required to work out the correct answers to problems involving a calculation and to do so without using a calculator. A pharmacist is expected to be able to perform calculations accurately without the use of a calculator. A pharmacist must be able to look at a figure and know that it is correct without any shadow of a doubt. These exercises will encourage you to develop and make use of various strategies for carrying out calculations and for validating the results. In making pharmaceutical calculations you can then easily draw upon the acquired calculating strategies.

There are many occasions for talking and thinking mathematically in the pharmacy surroundings. Look for patterns and relationships. What's your prediction of today's sales or of the number of prescriptions dispensed? How many different items are available in the pharmacy? What will happen if we reduce the stock of a number of items by 50%?

Attempt to validate general statements: Are the sizes of all inhaler canisters the same? Is it true that you cannot swallow whole a tablet that is 5 cm in diameter? Then relate your guesses to logical thinking. What makes you think that the pharmacy stocks fewer than 1000 different dosage forms? How do you know that tablets do not usually contain more than 2 g of the active ingredient? How can you be sure that your calculation is correct? Why can't you dissolve the calculated amount of active ingredient in the measured solvent?

In other words, practice answering these questions: What's your prediction . . . ? How many different . . . ? What will happen if . . . ? Are they the same . . . (size, volume, weight)? Is it true that . . . ? What makes you think that . . . ? How can you be sure . . . ? Why doesn't it work . . . ?

Finally, one last exercise to ensure that you are as familiar with mathematical calculations as surely as you know that penicillin is an antibiotic, is by practising drawing conclusions and testing them out. If the result of my calculation is that I need to give 1 kg of active ingredient in three divided oral doses, the chances are that I had better check my calculation. Simple examples of identifying errors would be: Is the answer a therapeutic dose? Are there preparations of that strength? A final useful mathematical check would be: Is the answer of the right order of magnitude? There is no better assurance for answering mathematical calculations correctly and passing this obligatory section than by resolving to think mathematically and numerically throughout the preregistration practice.

The same hints for the open-book examples apply to the closed-book questions. There were some factual points that proved more difficult than others. The following are some areas where candidates missed certain facts.

Prodrug:	codeine is a prodrug (T4 Q6)
Side-effects:	simvastatin may cause alopecia (T4 Q40)
	atenolol – mixing tachycardia with bradycardia (T4 Q78)
	clomipramine – may cause jaundice (T6 Q36)
Parasympathomimetic properties:	may cause blurred vision, avoided in asthma, act as miotics (T4 Q43)
Improper use:	aciclovir as a prophylactic for cold sores (T4 Q75)
	breath-activated inhalers less suitable for children (T5 Q76)
Classification:	chemical: furosemide is an anthranilic acid derivative with a sulphonamide moiety (T6 Q24)
	pharmacological: mitoxantrone is a cytotoxic antibiotic (T5 Q58). Micralax is an osmotic laxative (T5 Q89)
Labelling:	the term saline is an approved code used on single-dose eye drops containers to indicate 0.9% w/v sodium chloride solution (T6 Q80)
	Co-amoxiclav 625 mg tablets does not mean that the tablets contain amoxicillin 625 mg (T6 Q87)

Sequential questions (Test 7)

Test 7 consists of 10 questions of a rather innovative format. The logistics of answering these questions should be planned. Special attention is needed to identify the sequential order required. Scoring of the questions is usually developed to reflect a different weighting for each proposed answer. This system allows a wide variety of scoring methodologies. The scoring weighting may even vary from question to question.

Question 1

Putting in sequence the molecular weights of different substances is a common question. Usually it was common to ask candidates to match a series of molecular weights with different substances. This is a different version of the same type of question. The best way to try and reason out this answer is by placing the substances in accordance with molecular size. You can work out the molecular weights from the structure and the atomic weights. Organic molecules tend to be larger than inorganic molecules but this is not always the case, as in this example, where aluminium chloride has a higher molecular weight than glycerine. Knowledge of the size of a molecule is useful in pharmacy, for example, in predicting some of its physical and pharmacokinetic properties.

Question 2

A knowledge of probable reactions of substances could help a pharmacist to better understand stability and metabolic possibilities for a drug and in this way act intelligently in pharmacy practice, such as in determining storage conditions and in predicting metabolic pathways. Q2 investigates the candidates' basic knowledge of the sciences, which is essential in dealing professionally with a medical product. It touches on the principles of hydrolysis, reduction, oxidation, racemisation and intramolecular hydrogen bonding.

Question 3

Questions relating to the history of pharmacy and medicines have not been included in this text. However, Q3 is closely related to the subject and asks for the matching of the introduction of five classes of antihypertensives with the date when they were introduced on the market. The medicines concerned were introduced during a time-span of over 50 years, starting with the diuretics up to the angiotensin II receptor inhibitors. This question should be relatively easy for the literate candidate, except perhaps for the relatively short period of 4 years between the introduction of angiotensin-converting enzyme inhibitors and that of calcium-channel blockers.

Question 4

Pharmacoeconomics is becoming an important area of study in pharmacy. Concern over the cost of medicines has reached examiners, and pharmacists are expected to take the cost into consideration when dispensing medicines. Q4 relates to the relative cost of classes of antihypertensives. The answer to Q3 could serve as a hint to the answers in Q4 because drugs tend to go down in price as time passes, especially once the patent expires and competing generic versions of the originator product become available.

Question 5

The structure of a drug can help a pharmacist predict a significant amount of information. In Q5 you could classify structure B as a tricyclic antidepressant and whether a substance is acidic or basic, and hence the effect of pH on its solubility and the consequences of those properties, such as, for example, the passage through membranes. In Q5, there may be some hesitancy in deciding which is the least correct between statements C and E, where both are incorrect with reference to clonidine and imipramine. The correct conclusion may be reached by counting the correct parts and the incorrect parts in each statement. Statement C has two incorrect parts. Statement E has three incorrect parts and therefore statement E has a higher level of incorrectness of the two. At the opposite end of the scale, statements B and D are both totally correct. Statement B has two correct parts, whereas statement D has three correct parts. Statement D therefore has a higher level of correctness than statement B. A good way to attempt answering this question is by listing the results of the correctness in columns, as demonstrated in the table:

Statement	Correct parts (X)	Incorrect parts (Y)	(X − Y)	Classification
A	1	2	−1	3
B	2	0	2	4
C	0	2	−2	2
D	3	0	3	5
E	0	3	−3	1

Question 6

A proper understanding of terms is very relevant to pharmacy practice. Some terms have different meanings in different countries. It is important to be familiar with substitution regulations in the country where you intend to practise and are taking a registration examination. The statements in Q6 have been formulated to be able to be answered correctly, notwithstanding the differences in the exact definitions of substitution terms that may exist between one country and another. Some countries include the term off-patent drugs. This is because in some countries where therapeutic substitution is allowed, this may not be applied to drugs that are still under patent.

Question 7

As a follow-up from Question 6, a knowledge of bioavailability helps the pharmacist to make a sound substitution. Q7 intends to test a basic principle on the relative substitution of different dosage forms. A product has to go into solution before it is absorbed. Therefore the dosage form through which the active ingredient goes most quickly into solution is the one that shows the best bioavailability. There may be some rare exceptions but in such questions you should stick to that rule.

Question 8

Knowledge about the structure of the drug (*see also* Q5), as well as its physical characteristics, may give information about the classification of a drug and about its properties based on a knowledge of the structure–activity relationship. A slight change in structure can affect which receptors are activated or blocked, thereby predicting the activity, including side-effects of the drug by, for example, determining whether it is an agonist, a partial agonist or an antagonist.

Question 9

Pharmacists should know how to predict the pH of a solution of salts. The rule of thumb is to determine whether the salts were formed from weak acids or weak bases and strong acids or strong bases so as to be able to predict whether the salt solution will be acidic, basic or of neutral pH. A knowledge of the pK_a or pK_b is then helpful in differentiating how strong or weak the base or the acid is. It is also useful to consider the structure of the compound. In Q9 it is helpful to write down the structure of the carboxylic salts because this identifies which is the stronger acid, according to the position of the phenolic hydroxyl group.

Question 10

A good way to prepare to answer Q10 is to acquire knowledge of structure–activity relationships by familiarising yourself with the basic structures of the major drug classes and with how changes to the basic structure or to the functional groups produces changes in the properties of the resulting drug. Until this basic knowledge has been acquired, a helpful way of attempting this question is by writing down the formulas of a number of narcotic analgesics and identifying the missing cycle for each. Prepare a table as shown, which uses methadone as an example. You could complete the table using several narcotic analgesic structures. On completion, count the columns for each cycle and then classify the cycles, starting with 1 for the column with the highest total of missing cycles up to 5 for the lowest total.

Narcotic analgesics	Cycle not found in structure			
Example	Furan	Benzene-cyclohexane	Cyclohexene	Piperidine
Methadone	x	x	x	x
Total				
Classification				

Sealing a success

Whenever a tutor meets students preparing for a preregistration examination, they are either equipping themselves to complete the examination successfully in a very dynamic, exciting and challenging practice environment, or they are going in the opposite direction and are failing to acquaint themselves with the range of necessary exercises to gain essential capabilities.

There are many reasons why students go in either direction and the switch from inadequate preparation resulting in failure to an enlightened approach, whereby students equip themselves to succeed, does not come about by chance; it occurs through strategic planning. Often the switch happens, not because students have an excellent tutor or because they decide that it would be advantageous, but because they fail at an examination.

By serving as a mock examination, it is to be hoped that these tests present an opportunity for you to identify your own weaknesses and to take corrective action before sitting the actual examination. The tests should be regarded as a means of getting feedback and of gaining awareness of the experience needed to be successful. You should use the tests not only to calculate the number of wrong answers but also to look at the practice points that have brought good results – and do more of them. Be wary of using the results only to determine how well you are doing and resist the temptation to sit on your laurels if you get a pass grade in the mock test. You will not know for certain how you have performed until you sit the actual examination.

There are two essentials that need to be catered for to ensure success at a preregistration examination. The first calls for diligent and careful practice. You cannot expect to do well in registration examinations unless you have carried out pharmacy practice training sessions properly and thoroughly on-site.

The second essential is to set out a strategy of how to approach both the practice and the examination. Strategy is vitally important. Pharmacy practice has changed over time and so has the method of assessment. It should be kept in mind that a number of practising pharmacists were brought up, during their university years, and when in-service training was not as rigorous as it is today, on a practice diet of oversimplified, prescription-filling tasks based on the ability to dispense as many scripts as possible (albeit without committing gross errors) in the shortest possible time.

Pharmacy practice has changed over time from being solely product-oriented, and now includes patient orientation, referred to today as pharmaceutical care. These aspects of pharmacy practice are very well reflected in the examination assessments. An exceptional few pharmacy managers may be indifferent to such a situation. They still use practice models that are static; some are even irrelevant to today's practice, whereas others may even be outright dangerous. In such cases preregistration trainees should insist on changing their mentor.

There are no simple matrices or algorithms that can be used to prepare for this type of MCQ examination. You cannot devise easy matrices consisting of four or five steps to ensure a success. The methodology of setting rigid rules to groom yourself for examinations has appealed to students and academics alike for some time but it is no longer valid. The use of matrices may be of some use during academic programmes, for example to study pharmaceutical chemistry or mathematics, but the effective transfer from the classroom to the practice world is different.

It is this difference that you must be conscious of when approaching a preregistration examination (and during pharmacy practice sessions), as opposed to when preparing for the final degree science-based examinations. The practice world is a great deal more complex than some of the traditional guideline matrices, which are devised to be followed rigidly, as you soon realise during properly guided in-service training. The strategy needed to prepare for the preregistration examination is more complex than for a science-based one.

Behaving like a valid pharmacy practitioner, as if you were in an unsupervised environment, is the best guarantee for success. Working diligently through the tests in this book provides you with a mock examination and its analysis. This exercise can be instrumental in ensuring that you achieve a good pass.

Bibliography

Azzopardi LM (2000). *Validation Instruments for Community Pharmacy: Pharmaceutical Care for the Third Millennium*, Binghamton, New York: Pharmaceutical Products Press.

Brunton LL, Lazo JS, Parker KL (eds) (2006). *Goodman & Gilman's The Pharmacological Basis of Therapeutics*, 11th edn. New York: McGraw-Hill.

Como DN (1998). *Mosby's Medical, Nursing and Allied Health Dictionary*, 5th edn. St Louis, Missouri: Mosby.

Edwards C, Stillman P (2000). *Minor Illness or Major Disease? Responding to Symptoms in the Pharmacy*, 3rd edn. London: Pharmaceutical Press.

Greene RJ, Harris ND (2000). *Pathology and Therapeutics for Pharmacists: A Basis for Clinical Pharmacy Practice*, 2nd edn. London: Pharmaceutical Press.

Harman RJ, Mason P, eds (2002). *Handbook of Pharmacy Healthcare: Diseases and Patient Advice*, 2nd edn. London: Pharmaceutical Press.

Mehta DK, ed (2006). *British National Formulary*, 51st edn. London: Pharmaceutical Press.

Nathan A (2002). *Non-prescription Medicines*, 2nd edn. London: Pharmaceutical Press.

Pagana KD, Pagana TJ (1998). *Mosby's Manual of Diagnostic and Laboratory Tests*, St Louis, Missouri: Mosby.

Randall MD, Neil KE (2004). *Disease Management*, London: Pharmaceutical Press.

Rees JA, Smith I, Smith B (2005). *Introduction to Pharmaceutical Calculations*, 2nd edn. London: Pharmaceutical Press.

Royal Pharmaceutical Society of Great Britain (2005). *Medicines, Ethics and Practice: a Guide for Pharmacists*. London: Pharmaceutical Press.

Royal Pharmaceutical Society of Great Britain Education and Registration Directorate. From pharmacy graduate to pharmacist. *Pharm J* 2005; **274**: 774–775.

Sweetman SC, ed (2004). *Martindale: The Complete Drug Reference*, 34th edn. London: Pharmaceutical Press.

Taylor LM (2002). *Pharmacy Preregistration Handbook: A Survival Guide*, 2nd edn. London: Pharmaceutical Press.

Walker R, Edwards C (2003). *Clinical Pharmacy and Therapeutics*, 3rd edn. Edinburgh: Churchill Livingstone.

Appendix A

Proprietary (trade) names and equivalent generic names

Actifed Chesty Coughs	guaifenesin, pseudoephedrine, triprolidine
Adalat	nifedipine
Aerodiol	estradiol
Alupent	orciprenaline
Anafranil	clomipramine
Anthisan	mepyramine
Anusol	bismuth oxide, peru balsam, zinc oxide
Arcoxia	etoricoxib
Aredia	disodium pamidronate
Atrovent	ipratropium
Augmentin	clavulanic acid, amoxicillin
Avelox	moxifloxacin
Bactroban	mupirocin
Beconase	beclometasone
Becotide	beclometasone
Beecham's Hot Lemon Powder	paracetamol, phenylephrine
Benylin with Codeine	codeine, diphenhydramine, menthol
Betnovate	betamethasone
Betoptic	betaxolol
Bezalip	bezafibrate
Bisodol Heartburn Relief	alginic acid, magaldrate, sodium bicarbonate
Bonjela Teething gel	cetalkonium, lidocaine
Bradosol	benzalkonium
Brufen	ibuprofen
BurnEze	benzocaine
Buscopan	hyoscine
Calcium-Sandoz	calcium
Canesten	clotrimazole
Cardura	doxazosin
Celebrex	celecoxib
Cerumol	arachis oil, chlorobutanol, paradichlorobenzene

Cilest	ethinylestradiol, norgestimate
Ciproxin	ciprofloxacin
Co-Diovan	hydrochlorthiazide, valsartan
Colofac	mebeverine
Combivent	ipratropium, salbutamol
Contac	pseudoephedrine
Cordarone X	amiodarone
Coversyl	perindopril
Covonia Mentholated Cough Mixture	liquorice, menthol, squill
Cozaar	losartan
Cutivate	fluticasone
Daktarin	miconazole
Day Nurse	paracetamol, pholcodine, pseudoephedrine
Deltacortril	prednisolone
Dentinox colic drops	simeticone
Depo-Medrone	methylprednisolone
Dequacaine	benzocaine, dequalinium
Dermovate	clobetasol
Dexa-Rhinaspray Duo	dexamethasone, tramazoline
Diamox	acetazolamide
Differin	adapalene
Diflucan	fluconazole
Diovan	valsartan
Dubam cream	methyl salicylate, menthol, cineole
Dulco-lax	bisacodyl
Duphalac	lactulose
E45	light liquid paraffin, white soft paraffin, wool fat
En-De-Kay	fluoride
Eno	citric acid, sodium bicarbonate, sodium carbonate
Eumovate	clobetasone
Eurax	crotamiton
Famvir	famciclovir
Feldene	piroxicam
Femoston	estradiol, dydrogesterone
Flagyl	metronidazole

Forceval junior capsules	ascorbic acid, biotin, cyanocobalamin, folic acid, nicotinamide, pantothenic acid, pyridoxine, riboflavin, thiamine, vitamin A, vitamin D_2, vitamin E, vitamin K_1, chromium, copper, iodine, iron, magnesium, manganese, molybdenum, selenium, zinc
Fosamax	alendronic acid
Fucidin	fusidic acid
Fucithalmic	fusidic acid
Fungilin	amphotericin
Fybogel	ispaghula husk
Gaviscon Advance	sodium alginate, potassium bicarbonate
Gaviscon liquid	sodium alginate, sodium bicarbonate, calcium carbonate
Gaviscon tablets	alginic acid, dried aluminium hydroxide, magnesium trisilicate, sodium bicarbonate
Ibutop	ibuprofen
Ikorel	nicorandil
Imigran	sumatriptan
Intal	sodium cromoglicate
Klaricid	clarithromycin
Lamisil	terbinafine
Largactil	chlorpromazine
Lescol	fluvastatin
Levitra	vardenafil
Lipitor	atorvastatin
Locobiotal	fusafungine
Locoid C	hydrocortisone butyrate, chlorquinaldol
Losec	omeprazole
Maalox Plus	aluminium hydroxide, magnesium hydroxide, simeticone
Maalox	aluminium hydroxide, magnesium hydroxide
Maxepa	concentrated fish oils containing eicosapentaenoic acid
Meggezones	menthol
Merocaine	benzocaine, cetylpyridinium
Meronem	meropenem
Micardis	telmisartan
Micralax	sodium citrate, sodium alkylsulphoacetate, sorbic acid, glycerol, sorbitol

Migraleve pink tablets	paracetamol, codeine buclizine
Migraleve yellow tablets	paracetamol, codeine
Migril	ergotamine
Minulet	ethinylestradiol, gestodene
Mixtard	biphasic isophane insulin, isophane
Mobic	meloxicam
Mucodyne	carbocisteine
Natrilix	indapamide
Neoclarityn	desloratidine
Nexium	esomeprazole
Night Nurse	dextromethorphan, paracetamol, promethazine
Nizoral	ketoconazole
NovoNorm	repaglinide
Nuelin	theophylline
Nuvelle	estradiol, levonorgestrel
Nystan	nystatin
Ortho-Gynest	estriol
Oruvail	ketoprofen
Otosporin	hydrocortisone, neomycin, polymyxin B
Panadol Extra	paracetamol, caffeine
Pariet	rabeprazole
Persantin	dipyridamole
Phillips' Milk of Magnesia	magnesium hydroxide
Plaquenil	hydroxychloroquine
Premarin	conjugated oestrogens
Prempak-C	conjugated oestrogens, norgestrel
Prexige	lumiracoxib
Proctosedyl	cinchocaine, hydrocortisone
Progynova	estradiol
Pulmicort	budesonide
Remicade	infliximab
Rennie	calcium carbonate, magnesium carbonate
Rhinocort Aqua	budesonide
Risperdal	risperidone
Sanomigran	pizotifen
Septrin	trimethoprim, sulfamethoxazole

Serevent	salmeterol
Seroquel	quetiapine
Slow-K	potassium chloride
Sofradex	dexamethasone, framycetin
Solpadeine Max	codeine, paracetamol
Spasmonal	alverine
Sporanox	itraconazole
Stelazine	trifluoperazine
Stemetil	prochlorperazine
Stilnoct	zolpidem
Symbicort	budesonide, formoterol
Syndol	caffeine, codeine, doxylamine, paracetamol
Tambocor	flecainide
Tavanic	levofloxacin
Tenormin	atenolol
Timoptol	timolol
Tofranil	imipramine
Trandate	labetalol
Trisequens	estradiol, norethisterone
Trusopt	dorzolamide
Ultraproct	cinchocaine, fluocortolone
Uniflu	caffeine, codeine, diphenhydramine, paracetamol, phenylephrine
Utinor	norfloxacin
Ventolin	salbutamol
Vicks Medinite	dextromethorphan, doxylamine, ephedrine, paracetamol
Vicks Sinex	oxymetazoline
Vivioptal	biotin, calcium ascorbate, colecalciferol, cyanocobalamin, dexpanthenol, folic acid, inositol, nicotinamide, pyridoxine, riboflavin, rutoside, thiamine, vitamin A, vitamin E, calcium, cobalt, copper, iron, magnesium, manganese, potassium, sodium, zinc, adenosine, choline, ethyl linoleate, lecithin, lysine, orotic acid
Voltarol Ophtha	diclofenac
Voltarol	diclofenac
Xalatan	latanoprost

Xatral XL	alfuzosin
Xyloproct	aluminium acetate, hydrocortisone, lidocaine, zinc oxide
Xyzal	levocetirizine
Yasmin	drosperinone, ethinylestradiol
Zaditen	ketotifen
Zantac	ranitidine
Zestril	lisinopril
Zinacef	cefuroxime
Zofran	ondansetron
Zomig	zolmitriptan
Zyban	bupropion
Zyloric	allopurinol

Appendix B

Definitions of conditions and terminology

Adrenal atrophy: shrinkage of the adrenal gland leading to lower physiological activity

Agranulocytosis: a drastic reduction in the white blood cell count

Akathisia: a condition where the patient presents with restlessness and agitation

Albuminuria: abnormally large quantities of the protein albumin in urine

Allergic conjunctivitis: inflammation of the conjunctiva caused by an allergic component

Allergic rhinitis: hay fever, inflammation of the nasal pathways

Alopecia: hair loss

Alzheimer's disease: progressive deterioration of cognitive functions

Amnesia: memory loss following brain damage or trauma

Anal fissure: a tear in the skin of the anal margin

Androgenetic alopecia: male-pattern alopecia

Angina: thoracic pain caused by lack of oxygen supply to the myocardium

Aplastic anaemia: reduction in the blood count of all formed elements of blood caused by failure of the bone marrow

Ascites: accumulation of fluids in the abdomen

Asthenia: loss of energy

Asthma: a respiratory condition caused by constriction of the bronchi which leads to recurring episodes of paroxysmal dyspnoea and wheezing

Ataxia: inability to coordinate movements

Atherogenesis: development of plaques along the lining of arteries

Athlete's foot: tinea pedis, fungal infection of the foot commonly presenting between the toes and on the soles

Attention deficit hyperactivity disorder: condition characterised by poor concentration and inability to maintain attention, hyperactive state

Audit: assessment and evaluation procedures

Autism: a mental condition characterised by abnormal social relationships, speech problems, compulsive behaviour

Barotrauma: problem that develops because of exposure to increased environmental air pressure

Basal cell carcinoma: a malignant tumour in the epithelial cells of the skin

Benign prostatic hyperplasia: non-malignant condition caused by enlargement of the prostate gland

Bradycardia: heart rate less than 60 beats/minute

Bronchitis: inflammation of the mucous membranes in the tracheo-bronchial tree

Bronchoconstriction: constriction of the bronchi resulting in narrowing of the respiratory airways

Bronchospasm: acute narrowing of the respiratory airways caused by an abnormal contraction of the smooth muscle in the bronchi

Candidiasis: infection caused by *Candida* species

Capsulitis: inflammation of the capsule usually occurring in the shoulder

Cardiomyopathy: conditions that interfere with cardiac structure and function

Carpal tunnel syndrome: compression of the median nerve within the carpal tunnel which is characterised by pain in the wrist and hand

Cataracts: a condition where there is loss of transparency of the lens

Chickenpox: infection caused by the varicella zoster virus

Chloasma: skin pigmentation of the face occurring during pregnancy or with the use of oral contraceptives

Cholestasis: blocking of the bile pathway in the biliary system

Cirrhosis: a chronic condition of the liver that results in degeneration of the lobes and parenchyma and fatty infiltration

Cold sores: infection caused by herpes simplex virus

Congestive heart failure: a condition where the heart is not pumping efficiently

Conjunctivitis: inflammation of the conjunctiva

Cushing's syndrome: a metabolic disorder caused by excessive exposure to cortisol or corticosteroids

Cystitis: urinary tract bacterial infection

Deep-vein thrombosis: thrombus formation in one of the deep veins

Dementia: a progressive organic mental condition characterised by impairment of control of memory, disorientation and confusion

Dermatitis herpetiformis: chronic condition characterised with severe pruritus and skin lesions

Diabetes mellitus: a condition characterised by disorders in carbohydrate, fat and protein metabolism, which usually leads to hyperglycaemia

Diabetic nephropathy: disorders of the kidney associated with diabetes mellitus

Diabetic neuropathy: sensory and motor disturbances in the peripheral nervous system associated with diabetes mellitus

Diabetic retinopathy: damage in the retinal blood vessels associated with diabetes mellitus

Diuresis: increased production and passage of urine

Dysmenorrhoea: painful menstruation

Dyspepsia: epigastric discomfort

Dysphagia: difficulty in swallowing

Dystonia: impairment in muscle tone commonly occurring as excessive tone in the head, neck and tongue

Ectopic beat: impulse in the heart which does not originate from the sinoatrial node

Eczema: skin dermatitis of unknown aetiology

Encephalitis: inflammation of the brain

Endocarditis: formation of lesions on endocardium and heart valves

Epilepsy: neurological disorders characterised by recurrent occurrences of convulsive seizures and sensory disturbances

Epistaxis: nasal bleeding

Erectile dysfunction: impotence

Euphoria: an intense feeling of well-being

Eustachian catarrh: blockage of the eustachian tube with discharge

Extrapyramidal effects: involuntary movements, changes in muscle tone and in body posture

Extrasystoles: cardiac contraction resulting from an ectopic beat

Extravasation: seepage into tissues usually referring to antineoplastic agents

Gastro-oesophageal reflux disease: reflux of the contents of the stomach into the oesophagus

Gastroparesis: decreased gastric motility leading to failure of the stomach to empty

Glaucoma: raised intraocular pressure

Gynaecomastia: enlargement of one or both breasts in males

Haemolytic disease: increased rate of destruction of erythrocytes resulting in release of haemoglobin

Haemophilia: bleeding disorders characterised by a deficiency of factors required for blood coagulation

Haemoptysis: coughing blood

Haemorrhage: a large amount of blood loss within a short time span

Haemorrhoids: varicosities in the veins of the haemorrhoidal plexus in the lower rectum and anus

Haemostasis: cessation of bleeding

Head lice: parasites that attach to the hair

Heart failure: heart does not meet the requirements of the body and the pumping action is less than required

Heartburn: pain in the oesophagus usually caused by gastro-oesophageal reflux

Hepatic encephalopathy: hepatic coma, liver damage characterised by variable degrees of consciousness

Hepatitis: inflammatory disorder of the liver

Hyperbilirubinaemia: increased amounts of bilirubin in the blood

Hyperglycaemia: high blood glucose level

Hyperhidrosis: increased perspiration

Hyperkalaemia: increased plasma potassium level

Hyperlipidaemia: increased plasma lipid levels

Hypernatraemia: increased plasma sodium level

Hyperprolactinaemia: increased amounts of prolactin in blood

Hypertension: increased blood pressure

Hyperthyroidism: increased activity of the thyroid gland

Hypertriglyceridaemia: accumulation of fat as chylomicrons in the blood

Hypoglycaemia: low blood glucose level

Hypokalaemia: low plasma potassium level

Hyponatraemia: low plasma sodium level

Hypotension: low blood pressure

Hypothyroidism: decreased activity of the thyroid gland

Iron-deficiency anaemia: anaemia caused by iron deficiency

Ischaemic heart disease: diminished oxygen supply in the myocardial tissue cells

Jaundice: yellow discoloration of the skin, eyes and mucous membranes

Junctional tachycardia: cardiac rhythm that originates from the nodal-His region

Kernicterus: an accumulation of bilirubin in the central nervous system tissues that occurs as a result of hyperbilirubinaemia

Labyrinthitis: inflammation of the inner ear leading to vertigo

Laryngitis: inflammation of the larynx

Left ventricular failure: heart failure where the left ventricle is failing to pump forcefully enough to meet the requirements of the body

Legionnaire's disease: infection caused by *Legionella* species leading to pneumonia

Leptospirosis: an infection caused by spirochaetes that is transmitted through urine of animals especially rats and dogs

Livid striae: scar with bluish discolouration

Male-pattern baldness: baldness where hair loss occurs at the front

Mania: psychiatric disorder characterised by agitation and elated moods

Measles: an acute viral infection of the respiratory tract and characterised by a maculopapular cutaneous rash

Melaena: digested blood in stools indicating bleeding from the upper gastrointestinal tract

Ménière's disease: condition of the inner ear characterised by episodes of vertigo

Meningococcal meningitis: infection of the meninges caused by *Neisseria meningitidis*

Menorrhagia: excessive loss of blood during menstruation

Metabolic acidosis: acidic pH in the body fluids

Miosis: decrease in pupil size

Miotics: agents that bring about miosis

Motion sickness: a condition characterised by nausea, vomiting; vertigo caused by movement

Mucositis: inflammation of mucous membranes

Mumps: infection of the parotid glands caused by paramyxovirus

Myalgia: muscle pain

Myasthenia gravis: a condition presenting with chronic fatigue and muscle weakness

Mycoses: infective conditions caused by fungi

Mydriasis: dilation of the pupil

Myeloid leukaemia: malignant neoplasm of blood-forming tissues

Myelosuppression: suppression of the production of blood cells and platelets in the bone marrow

Myocardial infarction: necrosis of cardiac muscle

Myopathy: a condition characterised by muscle weakness and wasting

Napkin dermatitis: inflammation of the skin in the napkin (diaper) area

Nasal polyps: nasal mucosa that projects into the nasal cavity

Necrosis: tissue death

Nephrotic syndrome: renal condition characterised by proteinuria, hypoalbuminaemia and oedema

Neural tube defects: group of congenital malformations of the skull and spinal column commonly occurring because of failure of the neural tube to close during pregnancy

Neuropathy: inflammation or deterioration of the peripheral nerves

Neutropenia: a reduction in the number of neutrophils

Nocturnal enuresis: involuntary urination at night during sleep

Obsessive compulsive disorder: an anxiety disorder characterised by repeated thoughts and feelings of obsessions or compulsions

Oedema: accumulation of fluid in interstitial spaces

Oesophagitis: inflammation of the mucosa lining the oesophagus

Onchomycosis: fungal infection of the nails

Osmotic diuresis: diuresis caused by occurrence of substances in the kidney such as glucose and urea that will change osmosis in the kidney

Osteoporosis: loss of bone density

Pancytopenia: a drastic reduction in white blood cells, red blood cells and platelets

Panic disorder: an anxiety attack presenting with panic

Paraesthesia: numbness and tingling sensation

Paralytic ileus: decrease or absence of intestinal peristalsis

Parkinson's disease: progressive degenerative neurological disease characterised by tremors and muscle rigidity

Paroxysmal atrial fibrillation: a paroxysmal abnormal contraction of the atria

Pemphigus: condition affecting skin and mucous membranes characterised by formation of bullae

Peptic ulcer: loss of mucous membrane from areas in the gastro-intestinal tract that are exposed to gastric juices

Pericoronitis: inflammation of gum tissue around the crown of a tooth, usually the third molar

Petechiae: haemorrhage occurring in the dermal or submucosal layers, which lead to tiny purple or red spots appearing on the skin

Pharyngitis: inflammation or infection of the pharynx

Photophobia: abnormal sensitivity to light usually caused by dilated pupils

Pleural biopsy: biopsy of the pleurae

Pleural effusion: accumulation of fluid in the intrapleural spaces

Pneumonia: inflammation of the lungs often caused by an infection

Pneumothorax: lung collapse caused by collection of air or gas in the pleural space

Polydipsia: abnormal feeling of thirst

Polyuria: abnormal amounts of urine excreted

Porphyria: inherited disorders presenting with increased production of porphyrins in the bone marrow characterised by photosensitivity, abdominal pain and neuropathy

Postural hypotension: low blood pressure, which occurs when an individual stands up

Prostatic hyperplasia: enlargement of the prostate gland

Proteinuria: abnormally large quantities of proteins in urine

Pruritus: itching

Psoriasis: chronic skin condition presenting with red areas covered with dry, silvery scale

Psychomotor agitation: feeling of restlessness, commonly associated with psychiatric disorders

Psychoses: mental disorders

Pulmonary embolism: obstruction of the pulmonary artery by a thrombus or fat or air or tumour tissue

Purpura: group of bleeding disorders characterised by the occurrence of petechiae

Pyrexia: fever, elevated body temperature

Radial keratotomy: surgical intervention where incisions are made on the cornea to correct nearsightedness

Raynaud's phenomenon: intermittent occurrence of ischaemia in the extremities especially fingers, toes, ears, and nose commonly precipitated by exposure to extremes of temperature

Reye's syndrome: condition characterised by acute encephalopathy and fatty infiltration of the internal organs

Rhabdomyolysis: potentially fatal condition of skeletal muscle characterised by myoglobulinuria

Rheumatoid arthritis: a chronic inflammatory condition that has an autoimmune component that affects joints

Rhinorrhoea: production and free discharge of watery nasal fluid

Roundworm: worms from the phylum *Nematoda*

Rubella: a viral infection presenting with symptoms of a mild upper respiratory tract infection, lymph node enlargement, arthralgia and a diffuse red maculopapular rash

Salmonellosis: gastroenteritis caused by *Salmonella* species

Scabies: an infective condition caused by a mite, characterised by intense itching, which leads to scratching

Schizophrenia: a group of mental disorders characterised by distortion of reality, withdrawal from social life and fragmentation of thought and perceptions

Seborrhoeic eczema: chronic inflammatory skin disease presenting with dry or greasy scales and yellowish crust, which occurs commonly on scalp, eyelid, face, and ears

Sialolithiasis: formation of calculi in a salivary gland

Sudden infant death syndrome: sudden and unexpected death during sleep of an apparently healthy infant

Syncope: a brief loss of consciousness

Systemic lupus erythematosus: a chronic inflammatory condition that affects many systems in the body including skin, kidneys and nervous system

Tachycardia: heart rate more than 100 beats/minute

Tardive dyskinesia: uncontrollable facial movements

Tenosynovitis: inflammation of a tendon sheath

Tetanus: an acute serious infection of the central nervous system caused by the bacillus *Clostridium tetani*

Thrombocytopenia: a reduction in the platelet count

Thrombocytopenia purpura: a drastic decrease in platelet count leading to bleeding, petechiae and bruising

Tinea pedis: athlete's foot

Tinnitus: perception of sound such as buzzing, hissing or pulsating noise in the ears

Tonic-clonic seizures: a type of epileptic seizure characterised by a generalised involuntary muscle contraction

Toxic megacolon: life-threatening condition characterised by inflated colon and abdominal distension

Transient ischaemic attacks: cerebro-vascular insufficiency of a short duration

Urticaria: a skin condition characterised by pruritus

Varicella: chickenpox, a viral condition caused by varicella zoster virus

Varicosis: varicose veins usually in the legs

Vasomotor rhinitis: chronic rhinorrhoea occurring without infective or allergic component

Venous ulcers: sores that occur in veins that have been damaged, commonly occurring in the legs

Venous thromboembolism: blockage of a vein by an embolus

Ventricular arrhythmias: deviation from the normal pattern of heartbeat originating from abnormal electrical activation in the ventricles

Ventricular fibrillation: cardiac arrhythmia characterised by irregular rapid and weak contractions in the left ventricle

Ventricular tachycardia: tachycardia caused by consecutive ventricular complexes

Verruca: wart, viral skin infection

Vertigo: disturbance in the semicircular canal of the inner ear, which leads to sensations of instability, giddiness and rotation

Vitiligo: skin condition characterised by irregular patches that exhibit loss of pigment

Wolff-Parkinson-White syndrome: a condition characterised by disruptions in the atrioventricular conduction

Zollinger-Ellison syndrome: a condition characterised by severe peptic ulceration, gastric hypersecretion, gastrinoma of the pancreas or duodenum

Appendix C

Abbreviations and acronyms

5HT	5-hydroxytryptamine
ACE	angiotensin-converting enzyme
ALP	alkaline phosphatase
ALT	alanine transaminase
AMP	adenosine monophosphate
AST	aspartate transaminase
ATP	adenosine triphosphate
BMI	body mass index
CNS	central nervous system
COC	combined oral contraceptive
Co-careldopa	carbidopa, levodopa
Co-codamol	codeine, paracetamol
COMT	cathecol-o-methyltransferase
Co-phenotrope	atropine, diphenoxylate
Co-proxamol	dextroprophoxyphene, paracetamol
Co-trimoxazole	trimethoprim, sulfamethoxazole
CT	computed tomography
DMARD	disease-modifying antirheumatic drug
DVT	deep-vein thrombosis
ECG	electrocardiogram
FIP	International Pharmaceutical Federation
G6PD	glucose-6-phosphate dehydrogenase
GABA	gamma-aminobutyric acid
G-CSF	granulocyte-colony stimulating factor
GSK	GlaxoSmithKline
H_1-receptor	histamine type 1 receptor
H_2-receptor	histamine type 2 receptor
HbA1c	glycosylated haemoglobin
HDL	high-density lipoprotein
HRT	hormone replacement therapy
IMP	investigational medicinal products

INR	International Normalised Ratio
LDL	low-density lipoprotein
LMWHs	low molecular weight heparins
MRI	magnetic resonance imaging
NMDA	N-methyl-D-aspartate
NSAID	non-steroidal anti-inflammatory drug
ORS	oral rehydration salts
REM sleep	rapid eye movement sleep
SNRI	noradrenaline and serotonin re-uptake inhibitor
SSRIs	selective serotonin re-uptake inhibitors
TCA	tricyclic antidepressant
TIA	transient ischaemic attacks
WHO	World Health Organization

Appendix D

Performance statistics

Tests 1–6 were undertaken by a sample of final-year pharmacy students following a five-year course, which included the preregistration period. The percentage of students answering a question incorrectly is indicated for each test. Questions that were answered correctly by all students are not listed. For each test, the median score obtained by the student group is presented.

Test 1 (n = 24)

Median score obtained: 78 (range 57–90)

Question number	Students answering incorrectly (%)
1	4
2	4
3	4
4	8
5	17
6	29
8	33
9	4
15	4
17	4
18	8
19	17
20	8
22	8
23	8
24	75
25	21

Test 1 (n = 24) (continued)

Question number	Students answering incorrectly (%)
26	37
27	8
28	8
29	4
30	4
33	4
34	4
35	50
36	8
37	62
38	8
39	21
40	12
41	75
43	37
44	21
45	21
46	4
47	33
48	21
49	8
50	75
51	62
52	58
53	17
54	12
55	50
56	4
57	17
58	79
59	8
60	21

Test 1 (n = 24) (continued)

Question number	Students answering incorrectly (%)
61	46
62	83
63	33
64	8
65	25
66	37
67	4
68	29
69	33
70	87
71	33
72	21
73	33
74	8
75	46
76	17
77	29
78	29
79	12
80	96
81	4
82	8
84	8
85	12
86	37
87	17
89	25
91	8
92	12
93	8
94	12
95	17

Test 1 (n = 24) (continued)

Question number	Students answering incorrectly (%)
96	25
97	25
98	62
99	17
100	12

Test 2 (n = 45)

Median score obtained: 79 (range 66–91)

Question number	Students answering incorrectly (%)
1	4
3	16
6	64
2	4
9	31
10	38
11	2
14	16
15	2
16	9
17	2
18	7
19	11
20	2
24	4
25	42
26	7
27	2
28	22
29	7

Test 2 (n = 45) (continued)

Question number	Students answering incorrectly (%)
31	7
32	2
35	11
36	7
37	27
38	73
39	7
40	4
41	22
42	40
43	40
44	2
45	27
46	80
47	20
48	11
49	53
50	20
51	11
52	53
53	9
54	36
55	40
56	13
57	73
58	16
60	2
61	67
62	58
63	31
64	22
65	22
66	22

Test 2 (n = 45) (continued)

Question number	Students answering incorrectly (%)
67	51
68	18
69	4
70	16
71	49
72	51
73	69
74	89
75	33
76	56
77	13
78	7
79	7
80	78
81	7
82	4
84	7
85	7
86	16
87	9
88	20
89	2
90	20
91	11
92	9
93	9
95	7
96	71
97	20
98	9
99	2
100	38

Test 3 (n = 53)

Median score obtained: 75 (range 55–90)

Question number	Students answering incorrectly (%)
1	13
2	9
3	15
4	41
5	2
6	28
7	70
8	7
9	6
10	2
11	4
12	6
13	6
14	2
15	9
16	7
17	6
18	6
19	13
21	40
22	19
23	45
24	2
25	7
27	15
28	26
29	26
30	19
31	13
32	19
33	6

Test 3 (n = 53) (continued)

Question number	Students answering incorrectly (%)
34	4
35	30
36	32
37	32
38	6
39	21
40	87
41	23
42	2
43	2
44	41
45	64
46	58
47	7
48	17
49	24
50	62
51	4
52	15
53	30
54	17
55	85
56	9
57	15
58	13
59	11
60	11
61	41
62	68
63	77
64	41
65	34
66	38
67	23

Test 3 (n = 53) (continued)

Question number	Students answering incorrectly (%)
68	32
69	24
70	32
71	85
72	32
73	48
74	11
75	83
76	47
77	24
78	32
79	45
80	17
81	11
82	32
83	19
84	85
85	72
86	21
87	19
88	24
89	40
90	60
91	23
92	4
93	13
94	17
95	6
96	2
97	26
98	32
99	26
100	26

Test 4 (n = 24)

Median score obtained: 71 (range 62–85)

Question number	Students answering incorrectly (%)
1	8
2	33
3	4
4	17
6	79
7	4
10	4
11	50
12	33
13	4
14	25
15	17
16	12
17	21
18	12
19	62
20	4
22	4
23	21
24	4
25	33
26	67
27	50
28	37
30	4
31	54
33	33
36	46
37	21
38	21

Test 4 (n = 24) (continued)

Question number	Students answering incorrectly (%)
40	92
41	21
42	33
43	75
44	62
45	50
46	8
47	8
48	12
49	46
50	33
51	29
52	62
53	62
54	71
55	46
56	29
57	8
58	12
59	8
60	46
61	12
62	46
63	12
64	12
65	17
66	37
67	37
68	54
69	50
70	25
71	25

Test 4 (n = 24) (continued)

Question number	Students answering incorrectly (%)
72	12
73	58
75	67
76	58
77	4
78	67
79	46
80	46
81	17
82	25
83	17
84	46
85	21
87	12
88	17
89	29
90	33
91	25
92	62
93	4
94	21
95	12
96	29
97	17
99	12
100	50

Test 5 (n = 45)

Median score obtained: 71 (range 55–90)

Question number	Students answering incorrectly (%)
1	27
2	11
3	53
4	2
5	24
6	4
7	11
8	11
9	9
10	2
13	2
15	67
16	62
17	2
18	13
19	11
20	7
21	2
22	22
23	36
24	18
25	4
26	33
27	20
28	11
29	89
31	7
32	11
34	64
35	36

Test 5 (n = 45) (continued)

Question number	Students answering incorrectly (%)
36	20
37	4
38	24
39	16
40	78
41	4
43	44
44	13
45	40
46	49
47	69
48	47
49	31
50	64
51	11
52	38
53	13
54	13
55	69
56	4
57	56
58	89
59	18
60	49
61	56
62	16
63	71
64	22
65	71
66	27
67	13
68	38

Test 5 (n = 45) (continued)

Question number	Students answering incorrectly (%)
69	78
70	73
71	33
72	53
73	2
74	36
75	13
76	91
77	13
78	40
79	11
80	33
81	44
82	47
83	49
84	44
85	44
86	27
87	56
88	16
89	89
90	40
91	11
92	11
94	9
95	7
96	11
97	20
98	36
99	2
100	22

Test 6 (n = 53)

Median score obtained: 68 (range 43–85)

Question number	Students answering incorrectly (%)
1	28
2	4
3	60
4	28
5	6
6	7
7	7
8	4
10	7
12	21
13	4
14	32
15	57
16	4
17	13
18	2
19	4
20	30
21	24
22	30
23	17
24	100
25	6
26	11
27	53
28	43
29	2
30	2
31	2
32	40
34	51

Test 6 (n = 53) (continued)

Question number	Students answering incorrectly (%)
35	43
36	83
37	64
38	36
39	55
40	70
41	40
42	11
43	6
44	60
45	36
46	21
47	58
48	40
49	26
50	58
51	34
52	24
53	47
54	2
55	43
56	7
57	36
58	30
59	34
60	66
61	22
62	32
63	32
64	57
65	51
66	38
67	28

Test 6 (n = 53) (continued)

Question number	Students answering incorrectly (%)
68	21
69	23
70	58
71	41
72	2
73	66
74	23
75	13
76	7
77	53
78	4
79	30
80	74
81	51
82	42
83	40
84	53
85	32
86	4
87	74
88	51
89	55
90	34
91	55
92	19
93	21
94	28
95	23
96	79
97	53
98	32
99	49
100	34

Proprietary names index

Generic names index

Conditions index

Subject index